THINKING THIN

TOM **NICOLI**

KALLISTI PUBLISHING

WILKES-BARRE, PA

Kallisti Publishing
332 Center Street
Wilkes-Barre, PA 18702
Phone (877) 444-6188 • Fax (419) 781-1907
www.kallistipublishing.com

Kallisti Publishing titles may be purchased for business or promo-tional use or for special sales. Please contact Kallisti Publishing for more information.

Kallisti Publishing and its logo are trademarks of Kallisti Publish-ing.

10 9 8 7 6 5 4 3 2 1

Library of Congress Control Number: 2006936701
ISBN 0-97611115-2

DESIGNED & PRINTED IN THE UNITED STATES OF AMERICA

Dedication

To my parents, June and Tom Nicoli who have been supportive of all I've done since the start and from who's basic and solid philosophies I have built my living foundation upon.

And to my wife CJ and son Jesse who have sacrificed during my endeavors as well as supported me completely in all I've done. Without them I'd be less than I am.

And to everyone and anyone who has contributed to my emotional, personal, and intellectual growth for I have done none of this alone. I thank you!

Throughout **THINKING** THIN, you will find quotes that I found to be memorable. They aren't necessarily meant to be directly relevant to the text, but rather to give you things to consider while you are on your journey to becoming a better you.

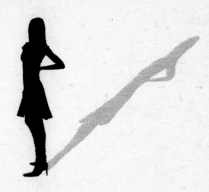

Table of Contents

You don't drive looking backwards...Stop living looking backwards.

— **Tom Nicoli**

THINKING THIN
ntroduction

The dangers linked to eating an unbalanced, fatty diet are not a secret — they are very well known. These risks are more documented than ever by many health and safety awareness campaigns. A large portion of the population is eating itself to death, piling on pounds and pounds with extra-large plates of chips, pizza, and other fatty foods. There seems to be no stopping this trend, and no limit to this global binge. The entire population of the northern hemisphere seems to have gone into food madness mode, leading to more and more heart related diseases, high cholesterol, and diabetes, as well as adding to the factors which favor the occurrence of cancer.

You know that, but when you get home from work tonight, you'll still probably grab a hamburger, followed by a big tub of ice cream. Even worse, you'll probably let your child have cookies, fatty meats and potatoes — anything that will satisfy their taste buds. You obviously don't do that to cause them damage, but that's exactly what you are doing. You're preparing them for a lifetime of eating fast food and putting on weight to an unhealthy point.

You know that overeating is bad for you and you understand that it will damage you and your children's health. You are basically doing something you know is bad for you and those you love most — and something that might shorten all your lives.

It might seem compulsive to you. It might even seem unbeatable. It's none of that; it's something you can change.

That's where **THINKING**THIN comes in.

THINKINGTHIN is a revolutionary new way to approach weight loss and to attain a fitter and healthier lifestyle. By utilizing methods and ideas that have been around for quite a while, you will be able to break yourself of your current, unhealthy habits and replace them with healthy practices that will enable you to reach your goals.

Diets, medical procedures, and the other sundry approaches to weight loss attempt to remedy the problem by working from the outside to the inside. "Watch what you eat!" "I'm gonna get lipo." "I guess I better hit the treadmill." These are the common refrains you've probably heard a thousand times (or more!). These phrases refer to things that are outside of ourselves — and are more than likely symptoms of an underlying cause. While watching what you eat will be essential to maintaining a healthy and fit life, taken to an extreme (which far too many people do) can lead to other problems without ever addressing the root cause of the imbalance in the first place.

You see (and you will see as you read through this book) that the root cause of your weight is not outside of you — it is inside. It is your mind.

How many diets have you put yourself on? How many pills that promised the fat would melt away have you popped? How many exercise machines lie dormant around your house?

Why do you think that is?

If you are mentally disposed to a certain way of thinking, then you will continually return to that way of thinking unless you aim to change not the behavior, but the cause of that behavior; and the cause of that behavior is the way you are thinking. In other words, you have to form new habits, which are nothing more than programmed ways of thinking.

Hypnosis (and self-hypnosis) can help you do that, by

making you feel that you can change it, making you realize that this is within your power, and helping your mind to take over from your hands when it comes to serving, eating, or helping yourself to food. Whether you are starting a diet or are already on a diet and find you are struggling, hypnosis can provide valuable help.

In all actuality, by using hypnosis or self-hypnosis, you are actually reversing the effects of the hypnosis you've experienced during your life that instilled your current way of thinking that caused your unhealthy eating and exercise habits. Another way to look at things is that now — finally! — you'll be able to take the reins and control what you think and how you want to feel about what you think.

That is the essence of **THINKING** THIN.

When starting a diet, hypnosis might help you to gain motivation, energy, and confidence, which are essential if you want to sustain the effort in the long term. It will make you realize that you really want to eat healthy, and, more importantly, that you can do it. It will also help you to remember every minute why you started that diet, and what you really wanted when you started it, which will help you stay motivated. You will see your weight-loss plan as what it is: a means to an end, and the key to getting healthier and fitter. It will remind you that it is not torture; it is not a mountain to climb. It is the opposite — the path of least resistance to a healthier life.

When you are already on a diet, it can be hard at times to carry on with the good habits. Festive periods such as the holidays, when everything seems to revolve around huge meals and decadent treats, can be discouraging, and you may feel like having a little lapse. Hypnosis will remind you of your objective, of what you really want. Even if you have a little lapse, this should only remind you that you need to get back on track in order to achieve the goal you set out to achieve: a fitter, healthier you.

Diets that suppress one or another category of foods altogether can be seen as particularly hard to keep over a long period of time. Many people report that diets drastically limiting carbohydrates are particularly hard to sustain.

Realize that cravings arise mostly when one particular kind of food is forbidden, and our minds tend to desire what they can't have. (In some cases, of course, the body may actually have been deprived of vital nutrients, which is why no one should ever begin a restrictive diet without consulting a qualified health care practitioner.)

If you are truly committed to sticking to a diet, hypnosis might help you to look at things in a more positive way. Instead of thinking about the carbohydrates you are craving, hypnosis might help you to release the creative cook in you and make more attractive, varied and appetizing low-carb foods. Furthermore, it might help you make the most of what you have, rather than concentrating on what you don't have.

And finally, it might help you re-focus on the goal you set for yourself when you started. By reading **THINKING** THIN, you will train your mind to act according to what you really want. Therefore, if your aim is to be thinner, hypnosis helps you to concentrate on that aim, rather than the means you use to get there, and whatever "sacrifices" those means might entail.

THINKING THIN is the revolutionary way to change the core, the true cause, of your weight issues. "Where your brain goes, your body follows" is something that we've heard quite often, but rarely does one grasp what it truly means. As you read, study, and practice the methods laid out for you in **THINKING** THIN, you will come to a true realization of what those words mean.

And you'll lose that unwanted weight in the process!

THINKING

TH[N]

Every thought therefore is a cause and every condition an effect.

— **Charles F. Haanel**

CHAPTER 1
THINKING THIN

Livin' Large

We are a nation of fat people — and we're getting fatter all the time. According to the 1999–2000 National Health and Nutrition Examination Survey (NHANES), a full two-thirds of American adults are overweight and nearly a third are obese. Contrary to what many people believe, there is a difference between the two. The definitions are based in the relationship between a person's height and their weight, typically referred to as the Body Mass Index, or BMI. A person is considered overweight if their BMI is between 25 to 29.9, while individuals with a BMI of 30 or more are considered obese. (See Appendix 1 for the BMI formula and a BMI chart.)

> As I ramble through life, whatever be my goal, I will unfortunately always keep my eye upon the doughnut and not on the whole.—**Wendy Wasserstein**

The Body Mass Index does not tell the whole story, though. In some cases it mistakenly pegs a person as "overweight" when in fact they are simply more muscular than the average person (muscle weighs more than fat). Furthermore, the BMI does not take a person's frame size into account. Finally, health and overall fitness cannot be measured by BMI alone; some overweight folks are actually more fit and healthy than their slender brothers and sisters. However, until something better comes along, the BMI is a good general guideline to help us determine our optimal weight. Like blood pressure and triglyceride levels, we ignore BMI at our peril.

As Americans, we've grown accustomed to the practice of spending ourselves out of our problems, and our approach to weight loss is no different. The weight loss "industry" is made up of all kinds of providers — from the old family doctor who advises moderation to the high-tech regimen du jour; from the latest fad diet creator to the manufacturers of "miracle" drugs that share one quality: the ability to make a sizeable portion of your bank account disappear. While there are many honorable, effective (in their own way) approaches, there are, sadly, far more frauds than miracle workers. Weight loss products and services in this country are big business, to the tune of nearly $40 billion in 2003, and projected to grow by over 5% per year to over $48 billion by 2006. While we continually strive to grow personally and to see our economy thrive, I don't think this is what we really intended. There are some kinds of "personal growth" we're really better off not achieving. The United States isn't alone in this phenomenon; obesity is also on the rise in other industrial societies the world over.

> Your body is the baggage you must carry through life. The more excess the baggage, the shorter the trip.
> —**Arnold H. Glasgow**

The flourishing weight loss industry is borne of twin parents: prosperity and our desire for instant gratification. Our very affluence seems to dictate that by eating ever-increasing quantities of rich foods, we are affirming that affluence — "I eat, therefore I am." When our clothes start getting too tight or we find ourselves wincing at the image we see in the mirror, we want to reverse the problem immediately.

You may tell yourself that you're not really that impatient, but ask yourself if you've ever stood in front of a microwave oven wishing your food would hurry up and get hot, literally begrudging the 60 seconds it takes to heat. When you add our ever-growing affluence to our impatience, it follows that we will spend exorbitant amounts of money in pursuit of an instantly improved image, even to the point of having excess baggage surgically removed or sucked out of our bodies — the quickest fix of all, and a multi-billion dollar industry in and of itself.

Those of us in the Baby Boomer generation can look back to our childhood for proof that obesity is on the rise. When we were kids, there was always the "fat kid" in any group, and he or she really stood out, typically being the only overweight person in the group. Nowadays, however, even our elementary school classes have a high percentage of children who are at least moderately obese. The one thing that hasn't changed is the way these obese kids are treated by their peers and even their parents. The "fat kid" stigma hasn't diminished even as the numbers swelled. (Sorry about the pun...sometimes I can't help myself.) They are still teased, often shunned, and held up as being role models for lack of self-control. The fat adults today can remember the teasing the obese kids suffered, and feel that pain as if it were a new wound. We certainly don't want to consider ourselves like the "fat kid" who was so taunted in our childhood, so as long as we can tell ourselves that we're just "big-boned" or "a little out of shape," we can avoid even considering that we may be fat.

In the next several pages, we'll look a little closer at the causes of our collective weight woes. Discovering the roots of the problem is the first step to finding a lasting solution. Then, by being truthful and honest with ourselves, admitting that we're overweight or obese, and committing to overcome the problem, we will have made a great start on the path toward a happier, healthier life.

How Did We Get So Fat?

The philosopher Lao Tzu proclaimed that the journey of a thousand miles begins beneath your feet. Thus does your journey to better health (and lower weight) begin by realizing where you are right now. Having eliminated an underlying physical dysfunction as the cause of the weight problem, we need to acknowledge the ways in which we have literally taught ourselves to be fat.

Those of us born into the Baby Boomer generation typically had parents who grew up during the Great Depression. During those bleak years, millions of people struggled just to get enough to eat, and learned to get food while the getting was good since they might have no idea where their next meal would come from — or when. While the inclination to eat more than necessary as a hedge against future famine is the result of millions of years of evolution, it was during the Depression Era that the "clean your plate" mentality became widespread. Just as people learned to eat all they could when it was available, their bodies also honed that primal drive to store nutrients against the lean times that were sure to come. These were pure survival instincts that served us well in times of need.

This mentality was further inculcated in us when many people decided to fight world hunger by airing commercials at all hours looking for donations and even by having donation drives or food drives at school. While these are honorable and noble deeds, this in turn caused many parents to quip at us when we did not want to eat any more food, "Clean your plate! There are children starving in (insert name of country here)."

Unfortunately, when the lean times passed, we weren't very willing (at least on an unconscious level) to set aside those behaviors. We found ourselves with plenty of food, yet were still compelled to clean our plates, no matter how much food was piled on them. And our bodies had learned their lessons well, and continued storing food away just in case the food ran out again.

At the same time, many people who had previously made their living by the sweat of their brow began working with their brain rather than their brawn. Our food intake stayed the same, while the amount of activity we did on a regular basis diminished. The end result is pretty obvious...we got bigger.

The hectic schedule that many of us follow is another factor in our ever-increasing girth. With so many different things to attend to during the day, we allow ourselves certain fixed times to eat — unless something comes up that requires our immediate attention. Then, we grab what little time is available, when it comes available, and eat what passes for a meal. Never mind that we might not even be hungry at our scheduled meal time, or that by the time we do get to eat, we're already cranky from the drop in our blood sugar level. We grab what is readily available — frequently a high-calorie, high-fat fast-food offering — and stuff it down as quickly as possible. If you've

We never repent of having eaten too little.
—**Thomas Jefferson**

5

ever seen (or been) a harried office worker sitting at a desk eating with all the grace and patience of a famished wolf, you'll get the picture. After our hasty meal, we return to what is, in most cases, a sedentary occupation, where we burn very few of the calories we've just eaten, and allow the fat to settle in…well…in whatever places gravity leads it. At least the wolf gets to run off some of the calories it takes in, and you'll never see a wolf eat when he isn't hungry! Now, if they had ever taken up wearing wristwatches…

The point is that we too often ignore our bodies' genuine hunger and satiety signals. We often eat when we're not really hungry (which, for most of us, is one of the surest ways to pack on unwanted pounds), or we fail to eat when we are hungry (and then overcompensate later). And far too many of us who do obey our hunger signals don't seem to know when to quit eating. We have to have "just one more" slice of roast beef or piece of pie, even though we're already so full we're groaning.

You might think that those times you don't eat when you are hungry would "make up" for the times you do eat when you aren't hungry, and that the latter wouldn't result in weight gain. For most people, however, it just doesn't work that way. The body stores the extra (unneeded) calories as fat, but it doesn't draw on those "reserves" when you simply skip a meal or two.

When you combine our learned, unconscious behavior — our bodies' evolved response to save up for lean times — and our "gotta do it right now" lifestyle, the end result is a "perfect storm" for weight gain, leading us to eat more and more, faster and faster, and pack it away for the famine that our body erroneously believes is sure to come.

While it may seem an indomitable task to overcome these conspiring elements, it doesn't have to be. We can't undo millions of years of evolution, but we can control our own behavior. Just as we have learned unhealthy behaviors, we can also unlearn them. And once those behaviors — and the underlying factors that reinforce them — are replaced with healthy behaviors, the tough part is over and a healthier and happier life begins.

Food: The "Cure" That Becomes the Disease

In the 1960s, there was a lot of talk in the media about the widespread "drug culture" that threatened to ruin the lives of a significant part of the younger generation. As it turns out, there was a lot of truth to the dire predictions, but it seems the focus was a bit too narrow. The truth is that the entire country has become part of a drug culture, every bit at risk as the youthful experimenters a generation ago.

> Gluttony is an emotional escape, a sign something is eating us.
> **—Peter De Vries**

We have become so accustomed to instant gratification, instant cures, and instant relief of our discomforts that we actually feel frustrated if one of our desires is not satisfied immediately. If we have a headache, we opt for a medication that works in fifteen minutes over another that works in thirty, even if by taking the faster drug we risk doing damage to our bodies in the future. All that matters is right now.

I briefly discussed the common tendency to ignore our bodies' hunger and satiety signals. Unless there is truly something wrong with a person's appetite control system[†], these signals are usually very

---

[†] Illness or chronic disease, pregnancy, certain medications, environmental changes, and even brain damage caused by trauma can sometimes cause the appetite control system to malfunction. Even in these cases, however, the problem can often be corrected with proper treatment, which may or may not include medication. Of course, only a qualified health care

reliable.

However, if we repeatedly ignore the signals and eat at the "wrong" times, we can upset this delicate mechanism. When it comes to eating, therefore, the real key to weight management for most people is not to follow a stringent diet, but simply to eat when hungry and stop eating when full. While this may seem self-evident, there are many factors, both external and internal, that make it incredibly difficult for many of us to follow this simple principle.

When we feel hungry, we will frequently delay eating until it is convenient or until we feel genuine discomfort, and then we rush to a fast-food establishment, where we get irritated if our food isn't delivered at the same time as we receive our change. Of course, were we to sit in a place of absolute silence as we ate, we would almost be able to hear our arteries harden from the enormous amount of fat in the food we were served. But that's okay...we were fed quickly.

And what about those "other" hungers that we so desperately — albeit unsuccessfully — try to satisfy with food? While the image of the depressed person eating an entire box of chocolates might be a cliché, it is certainly an accurate one. Or how about the self-described "connoisseur" who frequently relishes meals consisting of several lobster tails dripping with drawn butter followed by a difficult-to-pronounce pastry filled with custard and drizzled with cream sauce — only to end his day with prescription medication for his high blood pressure? The connoisseur might feel quite refined and sophisticated...at least until he has to undergo bypass surgery.

It is dangerously tempting to attempt to sate some apparently insatiable hunger with another more easily achieved activity. Can't find a fulfilling relationship with another person? Have a couple of eclairs. Feeling frustrated at work? Let the sensual pleasure of eating until you groan help you put aside those frustrations.

These examples are oversimplified and exaggerated, of course, but they are nonetheless clearly indicative of the common human tendency to mask unhappiness by engaging in some other satisfying activity. Many people try to assuage their pain with alcohol or other drugs — and many do it with food. After all, food is legal and it is easily available. And what could be simpler and more universally acceptable than to indulge in a glorious repast?

Naturally, food service providers would never try to discourage anyone from sampling their wares, even to excess. Have you ever encountered a waiter or waitress who scowled disapprovingly when you ordered enough food for two people — even though you were dining alone? Of course not! If restaurants wanted their patrons to eat reasonable, healthy servings, buffets simply wouldn't exist.† As you probably know, plaintiffs' attorneys and other factions have recently launched attempts to make restaurants and food manufacturers liable for contributing to our nation's obesity problem. For now, though, food is still the legal "drug" of choice for millions who are feeding something much more profound than physical hunger. Like so many other drugs, it is widely abused — and it is killing us.

Beyond the fact that we eat too much and often for the wrong reasons, we also tend to schedule our eating according to arbitrary events that have nothing whatsoever to do with our bodies' needs. Many of us are pressured into doing this, and we feel we have little choice. For example, factory workers will typically stop to eat at a given time, frequently

---

† I have friends in Texas who swear that any eating establishment that specializes in chicken-fried steak must, by decree of unwritten law, serve portions of meat that overhang the edge of the platter by at least two inches. (This is certainly not meant to disparage the great state of Texas or its residents, but rather to illustrate society's widespread demand for more food than anyone needs or can reasonably be expected to eat.)

announced by a buzzer or whistle, even though their bodies might not be clamoring for nutrition at the time. Eventually, the worker's body learns to expect food at that time and begins sending hunger signals in preparation of the meal. The "delicate balance" of hunger and satiety signals has been upset. Unfortunately, the mechanism that actually makes use of the food hasn't gotten the word that it is in need of nutrition, so it stores it away for later in the form of fat. The irony is that "later" never comes, as the body doesn't start using up its reserves until a serious state of malnutrition is experienced, and none of us is going to put off eating long enough for that to occur.

The flip side of this scenario is the worker who is just too busy to respond to hunger signals. "I have to get this (fill in the blank) finalized before lunch" is one of the most common mantras uttered in the business world. While we may be showing our employers and clients an admirable degree of loyalty by adhering to this credo, we are doing our own bodies a real disservice. Remember our earlier discussion about how our bodies learned to "save for a rainy day"? Well, by frequently ignoring our hunger until we finish some task, we are reinforcing our bodies' belief that those rainy days are indeed coming — and they react by saving up even more aggressively. That's why simply dieting is so ineffective. The less we feed our genuine hunger, the more aggressively our bodies work to store nutrients against threat of impending famine. Then, what little we do allow ourselves to eat takes the

> The second day of a diet is always easier than the first; by the second day you're off it.
> —Jackie Gleason

fast lane to our thighs, butt, and belly.

I certainly don't mean to imply that every overweight individual is a depressed loser for whom food is a desperate attempt to bring a degree of color into an otherwise joyless life. I hope I have made it clear that every one of us, overweight or not, tends to compensate for the frustrations we experience by engaging in activities that we find pleasurable. And while we might not schedule our lives by buzzers and whistles, each of us tends to allow outside events to affect the timing of our more basic activities, such as eating.

We are all on the same treadmill, to some extent. While we may never lead pristine lives guided solely by the needs of our bodies, we can at least begin to understand the harm our imposed schedules and misdirected hungers can inflict, and come to some kind of compromise.

With that understanding, we may begin to act consciously, steering our lives on a course that is both healthy and satisfying. The treadmills of our lives may always be there, but we can choose the pace at which we run, thus taking control, perhaps for the first time. By doing so, we can truly find the joy that has eluded us for so long.

> I've been on a diet for two weeks and all I've lost is two weeks.
>
> **—Totie Fields**

Past "Solutions" To The Problem

Sometime during the last couple of decades, we finally realized that more isn't necessarily better, at least where the size of our bodies was concerned. Our

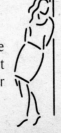

collective approach to the problem was consistent with our approach to anything else: hit it hard, make things happen quickly, and do it with as little personal effort as possible. As you probably already know, the only ones who really benefited from this approach were the pioneers in what was to ultimately become a multi-billion dollar industry.

Our earliest attempts at weight loss were pretty low-tech and straightforward: we simply starved ourselves until we lost the excess weight. It seemed to work for a while, though the experience was far from pleasant.

There were a few commercially available remedies available, such as candies that helped to ease the state of constant hunger and liquid supplements that made us feel full without taking in all the calories and fats that we were accustomed to; but these were really short-term solutions and failed to fully alleviate the suffering. I've even heard of some people who ended up drinking the supplements along with meals instead of using them to replace the meals. Talk about the cure worsening the condition!

Even as so many people were struggling to diet themselves out of obesity, they were ignorant of their bodies' natural reaction to their efforts. As I discussed earlier, we humans — like every other animal — adapted to our environment to ensure our survival. There were times when food was scarce, and only the people whose bodies were able to store up nutrients as a hedge against these periods of famine survived. As a result, with each passing generation, the people who could eat to excess — and therefore gain weight — when food was available would thrive and pass the ability on to their offspring. After thousands of years of this, the human body became very adept at packing on the pounds.

Nowadays, the "modern" effort to control our intake is no different to our bodies than was the ancient experience of famine. By dieting, therefore, we are literally encouraging our bodies to save up — even to the point of building extra reserves — at the expense of applying our food intake to the energy we need in order to function. We are literally dieting ourselves fatter!

It was only a matter of time before medical science would find something to help us lose our appetite, and thus, our excess weight. It was found that amphetamine-based "diet pills" proved to be immediately effective. When your heart is beating a mile a minute, the world is whizzing by at a blinding rate, and your mind is overrun with "brilliant" ideas, food is the last thing on your mind (with the possible exception of the chewing gum you devour so frantically just to give your body some way of using up all that artificial energy).

While the pounds definitely dropped off, there were a few "minor" inconveniences experienced by followers of this course of treatment. The first sign most people had that something was amiss was their inability to sleep. And when they did finally take a break from their wonder drug, they slept with a vengeance — and often awakened feeling horribly depressed. Rather than feel so bad, many simply resumed taking their medications, and found that the bad feelings went away — for the most part.

> You have to stay in shape. My grandmother, she started walking five miles a day when she was 60. She's 97 today and we don't know where the hell she is.—**Ellen Degeneres**

After a few of these giddy-depressed cycles, all too many people found themselves hopelessly addicted to these pills. Others began experiencing other little "inconveniences", such as heart problems, sexual dysfunction, and even paranoid psychoses. How could all this happen? After all, these people weren't street junkies; they were normal, law-abiding citizens and they had received their medication from their friendly family doctor, who would never hurt them. Unfortunately, the doctors themselves weren't adequately informed as to the downside of the medications they were prescribing. The in-depth studies showing the harmful potential just hadn't been done, and those that had been performed hadn't been widely publicized.

The more we learned about the damaging side effects of prescription diet medications, the more motivated we became to find more natural, "organic" means to assist us in our efforts. Not surprisingly, there was no shortage of entrepreneurs eager to satisfy the burgeoning market's demands. We were told that any number of naturally-occurring herbs and supplements could magically melt the pounds away, allowing us to continue to eat whatever — and as much as — we wanted. It seemed that a new "miracle" supplement was discovered every week, such as lecithin (which is, ironically, a significant ingredient in chocolate bars), sea kelp, and even grapefruit. Imagine our collective joy when we learned that we could gorge ourselves by day, then offset any weight gain just by eating a grapefruit at night! The entrepreneurs even went one better: they began marketing grapefruit pills, promising the same benefit without the "inconvenience" of eating those difficult-to-eat grapefruits. Great news, especially for people who didn't like the taste of grapefruit!

There was only one very minor drawback: none of these supplements actually worked to any significant degree. They only served to appease our need to feel like we were doing something, while our bodies — and the fortunes of the entrepreneurs — kept on growing.

More recently, we have seen phenomenal growth in the number of "health clubs" as more and more people begin focusing on exercise as a viable method to control their weight. You can't watch an hour of television without seeing at least one commercial showing young people with buff bodies and perfect teeth and hair, thoroughly enjoying their time dancing, kick-boxing, and aerobicizing their way to physical nirvana. I must admit, it's a pretty compelling picture, and the devotion to a reasonable exercise regimen is certainly beneficial to one's health. But what began as a means to a healthier lifestyle has become, in recent years, more of a social imperative than a health-related routine. Today's gyms have replaced the cocktail parties of our parents' generation, and the desire for physical well being has been replaced with an obsession for the right "look." It's not uncommon nowadays for a basically healthy individual to be looked down upon at the gym if they don't present the ideal body style — or even the "correct" gym fashions. As a result, too many people who follow the current trend as a means to improving their physical well-being end up even more discouraged than before they joined the gym and ultimately abandon the effort rather than feel as out of place as they did in their larger bodies.

> The rest of the world lives to eat, while I eat to live.
>
> —Socrates

On the other hand, we have those people who are successful at shaping their bodies so as to meet the "gold standard" of fitness. One wonders how many of them become so obsessed with the result that they never feel they have quite reached their goal. I've encountered a number of people who devote so much time to working out that they actually neglect other areas of their lives and end up feeling like hamsters on a wheel, unable to get off.

While these may be extreme cases, they do reflect the obsession with self-image that so many people have adopted, only to be frustrated. If you have struggled with a weight problem, you have no doubt tried many of the dubious solutions touched on in this chapter. It's quite possible that some of them were successful for a while, but sooner or later — probably sooner — you re-gained those lost pounds and then some. So here you are, right back where you started, perhaps more discouraged than ever — and perhaps you are blaming yourself and feeling as if you have failed.

If so, the first step you need to take is to stop the self-blame. If you want to place blame somewhere, place it on all those "quick fixes." You haven't failed; the "fixes" have failed you. They don't work in the long term for one basic reason: they are external approaches to a problem that needs an internal approach.

Fad diets, trendy supplements, and strenuous exercise routines address the symptoms, but not the essential cause of behavior-related weight problems. They don't even touch on the underlying motives that contribute to your weight woes. In a way, using these methods for permanent weight loss is much like punishing a child for errant behavior. Here I refer not to effective disciplinary methods, which as every parent knows are sometimes necessary, but rather to ineffective punishments that hurt, frighten, or humiliate a child. These may very well seem effective in the short term — for example, spanking a child may temporarily stop "bad" behavior — but eventually the behavior is repeated, or, at best, it lingers beneath the surface. This is because the child has been given no positive internal motivation for changing his or her behavior, nor has the cause of the undesirable behavior been addressed. All too often, the humiliating or hurtful punishment backfires on the parent and the child's behavior only gets worse — proving the ultimate futility of using external "solutions" for problems that need to be addressed internally.

Most of the weight-loss methods so many of us have tried are equally futile.[†] What it amounts to is that too many of us have been trying to change from the outside in, instead of from the inside out. We try to re-sculpt our bodies without "re-sculpting" our motives — or our self-image.

There's an old saying that goes "No matter where you go, there you are." Or, in the words of the late reggae superstar Bob Marley, "You runnin' and you runnin' and you runnin' away...but you can't run away from yourself." Unfortunately, this wisdom has been altogether ignored by the weight-loss industry.

If you feel fat and/or unattractive to begin with, it will generally take more than a change in physical appearance to change that self-image. In addition to shedding pounds and inches, you must shed the impression that you are unattractive before you can feel good about yourself. And if the path to improved physical appearance is one fraught with suffering and denial, it is difficult, if not impossible, to maintain the positive frame of mind so essential to feeling good about how you look. The good news is that you can turn even the most negative self-image into a positive one, but the change has to come from within. Certainly your self-image is reinforced by external changes, but the real work has to be done internally.

As a culture, we have literally dug ourselves into an unhappy hole, and too many of us are frantically trying to dig ourselves out of it, often using the same shovels we used to dig the hole in the first place. In my dealings with thousands of clients over the years, I have endeavored to help them not

---

[†] In fact, many of them feel like punishment for grown-ups; the "no pain, no gain" mindset seems to be pretty firmly entrenched in our culture.

only to reshape their bodies, but to reshape the way they looked at themselves and the world. I have helped them discover the happiness that I believe is every person's most inalienable right.[‡]

The techniques I have used are not new, not "revolutionary", and not "miraculous" — although the results sometimes feel like miracles. The health I have helped my clients to achieve has been not only physical, but emotional, even spiritual, as well. Well-being cannot exist without a sense of balance. The most physically beautiful person in the world cannot be truly happy without being in touch with a corresponding inner beauty, free of the burden of self-doubt and self-judgment that is so prevalent in our lives today.

In this part we've spent a considerable amount of time discussing "the problem" and only hinting about "the solution." In the next part, I will go into much more detail about what I have found to be the real solutions to the weight-management problems so many of us face. I promise you that by the time you have finished reading this book, you will have all the tools necessary to not only make yourself look and feel better physically, but to reshape yourself into the happier person you've always wanted to be.

---

‡ And I must say (in all appropriate humility) that I've been very successful in my efforts.

Thin **Thoughts**

Too often we ignore our bodies' genuine hunger and satiety signals.

The real key to weight management for most people is simply to eat when hungry and stop eating when full.

While many people try to assuage their emotional pain with alcohol or other drugs, many do it with food.

The treadmills of our lives may always be there, but we can choose the pace at which we run, thus taking control.

Fad diets, trendy supplements, and strenuous exercise routines address the symptoms, but not the essential cause, of behavior-related weight problems.

All problems and solutions are in the mirror of self-reflection.

— **Tom Nicoli**

THINKING THIN
CHAPTER 2
Your Body's Real Hungers

If you've picked up this book, hoping for a handbook that tells you how to really buckle down and lose all your excess weight in the next 30 days or sooner, then you might as well put it down right now.. You've devoted years to training your body to accumulate excess unwanted fat — however unknowingly you may have done so — and you simply can't expect to reverse all that "training" in 30 days or less and automatically maintain the changes. You most likely have tried those methods before and know that they just don't work!

Here's the premise: We are the most affluent society in earth's history with a standard of living beyond the dreams of most of the planet's population and beyond the comprehension of those living just a couple of generations ago. That's the good news. The bad news is that our butts, bellies, and thighs give clear testament to that affluence. To put it delicately, we are a society of fat people and that excess weight threatens to offset many of the advances science has made toward allowing us to live longer, healthier, and happier lives.

Granted, some people are obese as a result of genuine physiological dysfunction, such as glandular disorders and the like. For those whose obesity has a medical cause, there is no substitute for professional medical care. But these people are a small fraction of the obese population, and even they would almost certainly benefit from my approach in concert with treatment from their physician.

But back to the premise. First, how did we come to accumulate all the excess weight in unhealthy, unwanted stored fat? More to the point, how can we solve this problem once and for all? We must not be doing something right, because while we feed the weight-loss industry over $40 billion a year, we just continue to get bigger (as does the industry itself!). You would think that, being as how we're so incredibly affluent, we ought to be capable of spending ourselves thinner, trimmer, and healthier. But it just doesn't work that way, any more than we would be able to spend ourselves out of debt. We have to approach the real problem — to first understand why we're so fat and how we got that way. Then we need to address the real issues and fix the things that are broken, rather than inventing new ways to convince ourselves that they aren't really broken, after all. Not to imply that you are "broken", but it's the simplest way to make my point.

> More die in the United States of too much food than too little.
> —**John Kenneth Galbraith**

That sounds pretty straightforward and simple, doesn't it? Well, the solution is pretty straightforward and simple. The trick to getting the right answers, however, is to start asking the right questions. And that's what we haven't been doing to date. This book is my attempt to help you identify and clarify the factors that have left you "more" than you used to be, and ultimately, to help you reverse the behaviors that got you that way, without inflicting a bunch of pain, suffering, and guilt. The end result that we'll strive for is a healthy lifestyle and, by extension, an improved body and sense of well-being. We won't do it overnight, but by the same token, we won't be suffering in the process.

We won't be using any untested "miracle breakthrough" cures, either. We will, instead, go to the heart of the problem that drives so many people to unhealthy, negative behaviors. We will strive to understand the lifelong "programming" that we are each subjected to — some of it helpful; some very harmful — and will begin using proven tools to free ourselves from that which hinders our quest for happiness.

D.E.P.T.H. of Life

This is where my concept of D.E.P.T.H.™ comes in. I'm sure you've heard the saying, "You're either part of the problem or part of the solution." This may seem like an oversimplification (and perhaps for some global issues it is), but when it comes to you as an individual taking responsibility for your own life, however, it fits perfectly. If you have a problem and are not actively doing something to solve it, more than likely you are only making it worse. Most problems will not go away if you ignore them. If you put off making an important decision, you are still making a decision to do nothing. In other words, you cannot be an "innocent bystander" in your own life — you are either part of the problem or part of the solution.

> It is not length of life, but depth of life.
> —**Ralph Waldo Emerson**

D.E.P.T.H.™ is my acronym for **D**enial, **E**motional **P**ain, **T**ruth, & **H**onesty. It is a concise description of both the problem and the solution. More accurately, it explains the origin of the problem (whether it is overeating, substance abuse, gambling, compulsive shop-

23

ping, or numerous other self-destructive, self-sabotaging habits) and it also provides the key to the solution.

In our affluent, distraction-filled society, it is all too easy for most of us to live in complete denial of our core problems. And in this land of plenty we have so many ways to alleviate the emotional pain that results from not dealing with our personal issues responsibly. Stuffing our faces (for reasons other than physical hunger) is one of the most common ways. This often causes problems that ultimately make us even unhappier, so we "feed" our pain...and so on and so on. The key to escaping this cycle of denial/pain—deeper denial/deeper pain is to face our problems with truth and honesty. In that sense, you could also say that D.E.P.T.H.™ describes the journey from unhappiness to fulfillment.

D.E.P.T.H.™ has another meaning too — a deeper one, if you will. In order to make real and lasting behavioral changes we have to "dig down deep" and get to the root cause of the behavior. Externalized approaches simply do not work. Instead we must access the subconscious, for it is there that the "programming" (both good and bad) resides, and it is there that "reprogramming" must occur. This doesn't mean we have to spend years talking it out with a therapist, or sitting on a mountaintop meditating. In this book I will explain some simple and straightforward techniques to access the subconscious. You can do many of these yourself, and there are resources available if you desire outside assistance.

> Don't dig your grave with your own knife and fork.
> —**English Proverb**

24

Most of the information in this book is not new. The principles and the techniques have been around a long time, but in this society of inflated expectations and instant satisfaction, too many of us have forgotten them. I wrote this book to help you remember, and to help you put these principles and techniques to work in your own life. There might not be all that many truly win-win situations in life, but if you come along with me on this most pleasant journey, I think you'll agree that this process is, by any measure, a winner. For you will have taken responsibility for your own life — you will have become, perhaps for the first time, part of the solution instead of part of the problem.

Your Real Hungers

When you are struggling with weight problems, the first step in the "Truth" and "Honesty" part of the D.E.PT.H.™ process is identifying your "real" hungers versus your "phantom" hungers. By "real" hunger, I refer to your body's actual need for nutrition. Although overweightness and obesity are not always caused solely by overeating, most people who have a weight problem do have issues with food. Therefore, you need to begin paying attention to your behavior so you can figure out when and why you eat, especially when you are not necessarily hungry.

> Take twice as long to eat half as much.
>
> **—Anonymous**

There's an old phrase often used to admonish or ridicule someone who eats to excess: "Eats like a pig." What most people don't know is that, left to its own

25

devices and offered a healthy range of foods, a pig will eat exactly what its body requires. It is in the pig's nature to store food (a nature highly encouraged by breeders who want to realize as much body weight as possible from a given amount of feed), so the animal gets very large. Were the pig's genetic tendency to store surplus nutrients reversed, so would be its tendency to obesity, for the pig eats only for nourishment, unlike humans, who eat — and overeat — for any number of reasons having absolutely nothing to do with our bodies' actual needs.

Whereas the first step in our weight loss efforts is to acknowledge our present condition, the second step must be to identify what our bodies genuinely need in order to remain healthy. Just what and how much of each type of food the body actually requires is a constantly evolving standard, evidenced by the frequent revisions to the government's widely publicized and almost universally accepted Food Guide Pyramid courtesy of the U.S. Department of Agriculture and the U.S. Department of Health and Human Services.

You should realize that the Food Pyramid — or any oth-

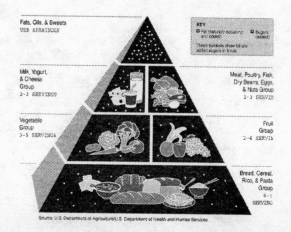

Food Guide Pyramid
A Guide to Daily Food Choices

er standard — is presented only as a general guideline. For example, a person who engages in a very physical lifestyle, such as a laborer or a member of a professional sports team, may require thousands of calories a day in a diet filled with protein-rich foods just to maintain even a minimum acceptable body weight. On the other hand, a person who leads a more sedentary lifestyle or who may have a slower metabolism might find that even a calorie-restricted diet consisting mostly of vegetable fibers causes them to continue to gain. Individual requirements, like individual body types, are unique. So how are you to know what is best for you? The logical answer is to first seek help from a medical professional, who will advise you about what your body requires and what should be eaten sparingly or avoided altogether. Believe it or not, your body can and will provide you with plenty of assistance in determining what it actually needs. We have all experienced "cravings" for foods that we don't normally list among our favorites. A person who is suffering from mild anemia, for example, might crave liver, when at other times they find the thought of eating liver distasteful. The trick is learning to identify (and respond appropriately) to those cravings.

> In eating, a third of the stomach should be filled with food, a third with drink, and the rest left empty.
> **—The Talmud**

Once your actual dietary requirements are established, then comes the frequently daunting task of modifying your intake to meet those requirements. As discussed in the previous section, however, there are many obstacles on the road to proper nutrition. One challenge many of us face when identifying genuine

27

hungers is that very few people have the luxury of scheduling their lives around their appetites. When we put off eating to complete some task, whether it is an important work assignment or a racquetball game played with friends, our hunger can get completely redefined. Where we might have been looking forward to lunch comprised of a spinach salad a few hours ago, putting off eating can transform our earlier desire for healthy fare into the desire for a fat-laden meal such as a cheeseburger and fries. This happens because as we grow increasingly hungry, our body recognizes the deprivation and changes the signals it sends from "I need nutrients soon" to "Feed me NOW!!" It wants something that will rapidly provide it with nutrients, even though the current object of its desire might not provide the long-term nutrition of our earlier choice.

Face it: a cheeseburger and fries or a super supreme pizza with everything but the kitchen sink on it rush carbohydrates to the system more rapidly and in bigger doses than would a spinach salad. Although the long-term health of the body would be better served by the healthier meal, the body has reverted to its age-old survival mode, demanding the kind of nutrients that will most quickly eliminate the "danger" it perceives. It then proceeds to store away a significant portion of the food as a hedge against future famine. Just by denying our body the food it needs — even for a few hours — we have reminded it that the "danger" of starvation is still real. This might sound foolish on an intellectual level, but we need to realize that it is based upon a cellular-level logic that helped us survive for thousands of years. Changing that logic and convincing our bodies not to react so aggressively isn't going to happen overnight..

While we're on the topic of real hungers, I think it appropriate to touch upon the use of drugs to control the appetite. I mentioned that true obesity sometimes may require medical intervention, which may or may not include the use of prescription drugs to regulate appetite and/or to normalize metabolism. Sometimes the appetite control system really is dysfunctional, and sometimes metabolic problems make weight gain too easy and weight loss all but impossible. These cases are relatively rare, however. Too many people have tried to use drugs, whether prescription meds or over-the-counter remedies, to do all the work of weight management for them. And far too often these efforts have backfired.

Many of us are familiar with the old margarine commercial that stated, "It's not nice to fool Mother Nature." Nowhere is the truth of that saying more evident than in the function of the human body. When those of us with relatively normal appetite control systems take medications that suppress the appetite, all we are doing is confusing the signals sent to our brain by the hunger and satiety (fullness) receptors in our stomach, and/or suppressing other receptors that tell the brain that nutrients are required. Eventually, the medications wear off or we stop taking them, and what follows is literally the body's panicked response to extended food deprivation. Our hunger rebounds with a vengeance, while our body goes into storage mode. This is why so many people find that upon completing a "successful" diet and losing the weight they desired to lose, they end up gaining all the weight back and then some — all in a very short time.

> Overweight and obesity is the second leading cause of death, killing 300,000 people a year... There is not a miracle pill that will lead to weight loss.
>
> —**Richard Carmona**

The goal in my approach to weight management is not to deny the body anything it needs, and certainly not to attempt to trick the body out of its genuine needs. Either of these approaches is doomed to failure, as anyone who has ridden the "diet and gain" seesaw can attest. Rather, I will teach you to genuinely listen and respond to your body's actual needs, not because you should, but because it will have become the most natural thing for you to do. For those of you who relish the self-torture and extreme discipline involved in dieting, I'm sorry, but you won't be getting that kind of "satisfaction" by following my program. What you will get is a return to your unique healthy weight in a reasonable amount of time, along with an improved general sense of physical and emotional well being.

In the following chapter, continuing these first important steps in the "Truth" and "Honesty" process, we'll discuss how to identify the pseudo- or "phantom" hungers we all experience, but which have little or nothing to do with our bodies' actual needs.

Thin **Thoughts**

We are a society of fat people, and that threatens to offset the advances science has made toward allowing us to live longer, healthier, and happier lives.

D.E.P.T.H.™ explains the origin of the problem and it also provides the key to the solution.

In order to make real and lasting behavioral changes we have to "dig down deep" and get to the root cause of the behavior.

Your body can and will provide you with plenty of assistance in determining what it actually needs.

The goal is not to deny the body anything, but to genuinely listen and respond to your body's actual needs because it will have become the most natural thing for you to do.

The thought is more overwhelming than the task.

— Tom Nicoli

CHAPTER 3
THINKING THIN

The "Phantom" Hungers

Whereas eating is a purely functional activity for the majority of the animal kingdom — or so we suspect, anyway — it is an activity that affects humans on many different levels. Since we derive pleasure from certain foods and displeasure from others, we frequently attribute qualities to food — and the act of eating — that have nothing whatever to do with nourishment. If you doubt the truth of this statement, just observe the expression on the face of a chocoholic as they bite into a Belgian chocolate truffle. Think that near-orgasmic expression is just their natural reaction to good nutrition? If so, please put this book down and contact me immediately, as I have a magnificent bridge for sale, and I'll make you a great deal on it!

> Forget love...I'd rather fall in chocolate!
>
> **—Anonymous**

We humans are very much sensory-driven creatures who tend to assign emotional qualities to our sensory experiences. There is nothing wrong with this tendency, so long as we don't let it dominate our actions to the detriment of our physical and emotional

33

well-being. As a matter of fact, many of our greatest pleasures are of a sensual nature. It has even been said that we
only fall in love as a secondary effect of our powerful sex
drive. Now, I wouldn't go that far, but it's impossible to deny
the fact that we make many of our decisions based upon
emotions, and many of those emotions are borne of some
positive or negative sensory input.

But let's get away from the science lecture and start looking at how these emotions affect our eating habits. First of
all, we tend to equate some foods with either a positive or
negative experience, and as a result, find ourselves either
craving the food or avoiding it. For example, some people
equate lobster with affluence, and if they aspire to a level
of wealth beyond their current circumstance,
they may crave lobster with an intensity far
beyond that which their
need for nutrients — or
even their enjoyment of
the taste — might inspire.
Somehow, the very act of
eating the lobster becomes
an affirmation of their level
of wealth and success.

> The biggest seller is cookbooks and the second is diet books—how not to eat what you've just learned how to cook.
> —**Andy Rooney**

For many people, sweets
represent the ultimate culinary
reward. The sense of satisfaction we
receive from cakes, pies, candies and the
like is hardly tied to the benefit our bodies
receive from eating them. What is it about these
confections that we find so compelling? Other than
chocolate, which some have claimed is actually addic-
tive, we would be hard put to identify the quality that
makes us desire sweets, aside from those times when
we deprive our bodies of food for so long that our craving begins to focus on an immediately accessible source

of energy such as sugar. On an emotional level, however, we have a completely different situation.

As noted in an earlier chapter, many of us who grew up in the Baby Boomer generation had parents who had lived through the Great Depression. Whereas our generation and those that followed view the availability of food as a given — an inalienable right — our parents had experienced true hunger and learned to view eating as a cherished privilege. Since it is difficult, if not impossible, to grow up in a household and not adopt to some degree the values of our parents, we brought forward the "clean your plate" mentality, which was somehow supposed to alleviate the starving of children in some far-off country. This was reinforced by adding on yet another emotional element: food as reward and/or punishment. We were told that we wouldn't get our cake until we ate all our broccoli. What this taught us was that cake was a reward for good behavior, while broccoli represented an unpleasant task to be completed as payment for our reward. While this was a simple means of enforcing healthier eating in children, in the long run it taught the children that sweets were good and broccoli was bad.

Unfortunately, we tend to carry these childhood lessons into our adult life, and these lessons guide some of our adult behavior with values that just no longer have merit. When we feel "punished" by some aspect of our life, we tend to seek out some reward to offset our unhappiness. Conversely, when we feel we've gotten some undeserved reward, we might be inclined to deprive ourselves of something that resembles a reward. We are, in essence, sending ourselves to bed without any supper.

Okay, don't go getting all huffy and start blaming your parents for that spare tire you are carrying. As we'll discuss later in the book, blame only gives rise to more dissatisfaction, which inspires us to seek out even more "instant happiness." If you're an adult, the responsibility for your actions is entirely your own.[†]

In many cases, when we are frustrated in other areas of our lives, we tend to seek out those simple, easily obtained pleasures we discovered as children. We also tend to rationalize. Had a tough day? You deserve a banana split. So what if it's too close to dinner? You're a grown up and can decide what to eat. And then there is the king of all dieters' rationalizations: "If I get the small steak, I can have the baked potato — and an eclair for dessert. And if I skip lunch altogether, I can go all out and have the 24-ounce ribeye — with all the trimmings, of course!"

It is our nature to desire happiness, but lacking happiness and peace of mind, we will frequently settle for whatever pleasure we can come by most readily. Although some of those pleasures are harmless enough, others can put us on the fast track to fatal diseases or the breakdown of our bodies.

> Your stomach shouldn't be a waist basket.
>
> **—Anonymous**

By now you probably have a pretty good idea about the ways many of us are driven by our emotional hungers. But there are other influences that have as great or an even greater effect on our eating habits. Those influences can be summarized as "life in the twenty-first century." In the previous section I talked about the fact that our schedules sometimes make it difficult

---

† There are, however, exceptions. If you are an adult, and your parents are still sitting there at the dinner table, arms crossed and demanding that you finish your dinner before you get dessert, there are a few other issues that need to be dealt with before we can even think about weight management!

for us to "eat when we're hungry, and stop when we're full." Let's take a closer look at some of the situations many of us face on a daily basis.

Say it's three o'clock in the afternoon and your department has just wrapped up a tough project. The department head invites all of you to happy hour at the local watering hole — her treat. You knock off early and head to the neighborhood pub, which is known for its happy hour extravaganzas. You have just downed half a cold beer when your stomach reminds you that you skipped lunch to complete the project. And there, not twenty feet away, is a table covered with those big food warmers, the aroma beckoning you. You stealthily approach your prey, not wanting to be obvious about how famished you are. Lifting the lid on the first tray, you behold a veritable mountain of those little weenies, floating in tangy sauce. You load up your plate (unhappy that the proprietor has set out such small plates) and go to the next warmer, which is filled to capacity with some kind of little cheese-filled pastries. You are pleased with your ingenuity as you fill your napkin with the little morsels and head back to the table. When you are through and no longer hungry, the feeling in your gut informs you that you've just eaten about two pounds of fat. But it tasted so good at the time and, after all, you were just being sociable. It's okay, though, because you will forego the dinner you had planned to make for yourself.

Or what about the friends who come over to watch the football game with you? You've prepared a tray of fresh vegetables and dip for everyone to share. They politely nibble at your offering, but unbeknownst to you, a couple of them have decided to be nice and spring for some "real" food — a giant pizza with everything you can imagine on it. Naturally, not wanting to offend anybody, you dig right in. Besides, the pizza does go awfully well with the beer...

These are but a couple of examples of social circumstances that can pressure us to eat when we aren't hungry or to eat something that we might normally want to avoid. In reality, our friends would rarely think badly of us for declining their offerings or opting not to join them, but it is frequently our nature to take the path of least resistance when we are included in others' plans. It certainly isn't that our friends and acquaintances are bad, or even that their choices are necessarily unwise. Quite the opposite! Our friends include us because they appreciate us and the food they provide should be viewed as a gift.[†] We need to learn to respond to our own appetites, rather than the appetites of others and to (graciously) decline the opportunities to sate a hunger that we don't feel.

What we need most is to learn how to reclaim the power to make good decisions for ourselves, rather than basing our decisions on unconscious issues or outside influences. We need to realize that an extra helping of pie won't make us feel better about ourselves and our lives, and that our true friendships aren't founded solely upon our willingness to eat the same things as our friends, especially when we don't feel hungry. And that is the focus of the next chapter: Robbing the "phantoms" of their power.

[†] The exceptions are those "friends" who have been continually resistant to our efforts to eat a healthier diet and have repeatedly tried to tempt us away from our commitment. These "friends" are best viewed as the human equivalent of "bad" cholesterol and avoided entirely.

Thin **Thoughts**

We frequently attribute qualities to food — and the act of eating — that have nothing whatsoever to do with nourishment.

We humans are very much sensory-driven creatures who tend to assign emotional qualities to our sensory experiences.

When we feel "punished" by some aspect of our life, we tend to seek out some reward to offset our unhappiness.

We need to learn to respond to our own appetites, rather than the appetites of others and to decline the opportunities to sate a hunger that we don't feel.

All goals are achieved in steps. Break down the main goal into smaller goals and see how easy it becomes.

— **Tom Nicoli**

CHAPTER 4
THINKING THIN

Exorcising the "Phantoms"

In this chapter, we will begin looking at how we can minimize or, better yet, completely neutralize both the outer and inner forces that drive us to eat more than our bodies can use. In the last chapter, we touched upon a few examples of those "phantoms" and, hopefully, you've begun thinking about the various factors that have influenced your own eating habits. Once we begin to look at and understand the phantoms, we need to be careful not to fall into the seductive trap of blaming ourselves or anyone else.

The Blame Game

There's been a lot of complaining in recent years about the tendency in our culture to blame someone or some "trauma" for one's problems instead of taking personal responsibility. The conservative radio talk-show hosts in particular just love to go on and on about this (at least, until their own "feet of clay" are revealed), and many of us nod our heads in agreement. Well, we've done a good job of identifying this particular problem, but in our day-to-day lives, many of us are still playing the blame game. If you are serious about managing your weight, or making any lasting change in your life, you have to stop blaming. Sure, Mom and Dad made you clean your plate even when you were no longer hungry, but they weren't trying to manipulate or harm you. They were really doing their best to protect you from the hardships they had faced. Even though the hardships may no longer exist, their actions were based upon their experiences — so cut them some slack.[†]

Nor does it do any good to try and blame your friends who are always tempting you with fattening foods. After all, eating is very much a social event in our society, and the act of breaking bread with friends is a bonding ritual that pre-dates modern society. In some cultures, the sharing of a meal with someone is a sacred act. I have friends down South who would never dream of welcoming a guest in their home with-out feeding them, even if the visit occurred nowhere near meal time. These are loving gestures and should be accepted as such. The trick is to accept the gesture without engaging in acts of gluttony!

> In the Middle Ages, they had guillotines, stretch racks, whips and chains. Nowadays, we have a much more effective torture device called the bathroom scale.
> —**Stephen Phillips**

Perhaps more harmful than our ten-dency to blame others for contributing to our prob-lems is our insistence upon blaming ourselves when we face a challenge. Self-blame, as we will discuss momentarily, is not at all the same thing as responsibility. The latter is constructive and necessary; the former is destruc-tive and totally unnecessary — but, unfortunately, all too common. For those who are obese or overweight, the tendency to blame themselves is frequently reinforced by the attitudes of others. Obese people in particular suffer the slings and arrows of our society's deeply ingrained

---

† If you're a member of a younger generation, I'm sure you could still find some way to blame your parents for your weight problems — the trauma of their divorce; your hard life as a latchkey child; or any of the plethora of talk show topics we've heard about ad nauseum. If so, I'll tell you the same thing I'm telling the Baby Boomers: "Get over it already!"

prejudices, frequently turning these prejudices inward. The obese are too often viewed as weak, slovenly, and lacking in will power. Perhaps the unenlightened people who hold these prejudices are unaware of how clearly they show their disdain. In some rare instances, they may actually be unaware of how hurtful their "subtle" comments and displeased looks can be to an obese person. Or perhaps they just don't care. The end result is that the obese person usually feels — and is hurt by — their judgment. In more cases than not, he or she feels on some level that the judgments are warranted and the disdain appropriate. Too often this results in attempts to dull the pain with the one thing that gives instant pleasure: food. The cycle continues as the obese person grows fatter and the prejudices are reinforced.

To a less dramatic extent, the same dynamics apply to many people who are merely overweight. In our "thin-centric" society, even minimal overweight is often accompanied by shame and self-blame. Ironically, in contrast to the reality of increasing obesity, thinness remains the ideal. It's become so bad that we are seeing eating disorders such as anorexia nervosa and bulimia in eight-year-old girls!

It's Not Your Fault; It's Your Responsibility

To whom will fall the responsibility for breaking the cycle? Will the ignorant be instantly and magically educated? I hardly think so. Will the obese and overweight somehow awaken to a slender, svelte body? Not in this millennium. The key element in resolving the problems facing people who are struggling with weight issues is a single word: responsibility. Though it serves no constructive purpose to blame anyone — including yourself — for the situations in which you find yourself, you can certainly begin to assume responsibility for the way you react to those situations.

While many of the challenges we face are visible on the

surface, many are hidden away in the lessons we learned throughout our lives. It is these phantoms that pose the greatest challenge to our sense of well being. After all, being called a derogatory name doesn't hurt unless, on some level, you believe the label to be accurate. It is hard enough to recognize our own deep-seated prejudices against others, much less the judgments we make regarding ourselves, but that is exactly what we must do if we are ever to develop a true immunity to hurtful, hateful behavior. Rather than spend years (and many thousands of dollars) in therapy, striving to learn the core of your dysfunctions, I have found a series of exercises that will enable you to fully perceive, develop, and appreciate your strengths and positive qualities. By doing so, the petty judgments of others will wither to insignificance, and the destructive habits you learned in that most subtle school of childhood will be overcome.

In short, you will give yourself permission to act in a manner that is physically and emotionally nurturing, no matter how stringently you have denied yourself in the past. I'm not talking about some new-fangled miracle program; nor am I suggesting anybody embark upon some self-denying spiritual path. On the contrary, the methods I have used with such great success thousands of times, and which I hope to teach you, have literally been around for thousands of years, and called by a number of names. The fundamental goal has always been the same, however: to give yourself permission to be joyous and healthy, and to help you become intimately familiar with that part of you that is strong, compassionate, and wise. By building strength, you will make yourself immune to being injured by the actions of others. By learning compassion, you will find yourself striving to shore up the weaknesses you see in yourself and others, rather than needing to use those weaknesses to attack. And with wisdom comes the ability to set a true course in your own life, to follow it around the difficult places, guided always by a true and unfettered vision.

If all this sounds grandiose and unattainable, or even too darn difficult, I assure you that it is not. There is no requirement that you have a genius-level intellect, and no demands that you practice some complicated spiritual process. On the contrary, my approach is simple and straightforward, and requires no specific set of beliefs. You only need to try — to make an honest effort with an open mind. If you can do that, I guarantee that you will see a marked improvement in your appearance, in your health, and in your life. It won't all happen overnight, but you will start to realize the benefits almost immediately.

What Motivates Us to Lose Weight and Why

You may be thinking, "Could anyone who bought this book possibly not know why he or she wants to lose weight?" This, however, isn't just about motivation for losing weight, but rather about the motivation for making changes in your life, because — barring some physiological dysfunction — being overweight or obese is pretty much the result of a set of behaviors. Merely addressing the behaviors is only a temporary fix at best. To really correct the problem, we must address what it is about us that causes those behaviors. It's less about the motivation to not eat than about the motivation to be happy.

> The one way to get thin is to re-establish a purpose in life.
> —**Cyril Connolly**

I decided to wait until this point in the book to really get into this because most people trying to lose weight perceive that effort as being enough of a challenge. To suggest that they might need to re-examine their whole outlook on life would send a good number of them running in search of a simpler and less intimidating method. While I understand this mindset, I also find it frustrating, because the methods I use are neither difficult nor intimidating — certainly less so than the act of depriving yourself that is at the core of most weight control programs.

On the surface, the things that drive people to lose or control their weight are pretty obvious. We know that carrying too much excess weight is dangerous to our physical health, and in the last few years we've become much more aware of — and motivated by — health concerns. We know how much more quickly we tire when engaging in physical activities if we're carrying a bunch of extra pounds. And given the benchmarks that the media set for what constitutes attractiveness, pretty much all of us get the message that we're at least a few degrees short of the ideal to which we would aspire. We all want to feel that we're attractive and that we fit in with our chosen peer group, so we make an effort to at least resemble the physical ideal that is presented to us.

> Don't go out of your weigh to please anyone but yourself.
> —**Anonymous**

Going a little deeper, we touch upon even more powerful motivators, some of which we never consciously think about, and a few of which may seem impossible to satisfy. Going back to the "fat kid" we discussed earlier, we remember the kind of taunting and teasing that child faced. We might have even joined in on the taunting. And now that we're all grown up and have put on a few pounds, we find ourselves in an altogether uncomfortable situation, because now we have become that "fat kid." Even if we don't actually think of that child, we remember the taunts, or at least the attitudes — some of them our own — behind the taunts. It follows that we would apply those same cruel, judgmental attitudes to our new and bigger self. And if you think it's difficult to talk someone else out of their long-held feelings, wait until you try and talk yourself out of your own deep-seated beliefs! So here you are, a grown up "fat kid" calling yourself names and holding yourself pretty much in disdain. It's human nature and part of your survival instinct to reject negative thoughts about yourself, and your only defenses are denial and/or suppressing those thoughts. So you shove them deeper inside. They're no longer on the surface, where you can feel the pain they cause, but they are operating full-steam in your unconscious, leading you to do things in an effort to get rid of them altogether. Unfortunately, as an overweight person plagued by feeling badly about yourself, you might be tempted to seek some kind of pleasurable feeling wherever you can find it — like in a box of Ding Dongs™†. And the cycle continues to feed upon itself.

Face it. We've really turned into a pretty mean species. Even if we're kind and compassionate to other people, we have a tendency to treat ourselves pretty poorly. Ultimately, the purpose of this book is to teach you how to become your own best friend, rather than your own worst enemy, and to act in a manner that makes your life better, rather than adding pain to it. Maybe we would all be better off if the Golden Rule were expanded to read, "Do unto others — and yourself — as you would have others do unto you." If we truly lived by such a credo, there would be far fewer fat kids (and fat kids

---

† It is not my intention to selectively disparage any confection, many of which I personally enjoy. Ding Dongs™ are presented here as a metaphor for any seductively delicious treat that we fat kids tend to abuse. So please send your lawyers after someone else.

in grown up bodies) running around, and those who were left would have a much better shot at living happy lives.

As I mentioned at the beginning of this chapter, merely addressing the set of behaviors leading to your weight problem is not enough. We have to get to the root cause of these behaviors, and the only way to do that is through the subconscious. And that is what we are going to explore in the chapters that follow.

Thin **Thoughts**

Though it serves no constructive purpose to blame anyone — including yourself — for the situations in which you find yourself, you can certainly begin to assume responsibility for the way you react to those situations.

It's less about the motivation to not eat than about the motivation to be happy.

Ultimately, the purpose of this book is to teach you how to become your own best friend, rather than your own worst enemy, and to act in a manner that makes your life better, rather than adding pain to it.

Do unto others — and yourself — as you would have others do unto you.

TOM **NICOLI**

Everything in your life either enhances you or diminishes you — the trick is in telling which is which.

— **Tom Nicoli**

CHAPTER 5
THINKING THIN

Hypnosis and Self Hypnosis

In previous chapters, I've hinted at the methods I have used with great success for a number of years, but just in case you hadn't noticed, I didn't come right out and tell you what those methods were. I wasn't trying to be sneaky. I just wanted you to get a sense of what was possible before I even mentioned a word that is wrought with myths and misconceptions. That word is **hypnosis**.

Far too many people view hypnosis with the same wary eye that they would cast upon voodoo or black magic. Given the way hypnosis has been presented, such archaic attitudes are no big surprise. Ask the average person what his or her experience with hypnosis has been, and you'll likely hear tales of hilarious (if embarrassing) nightclub acts or memories of movies wherein a "mad scientist" would subvert some innocent to his evil will. The plot usually has the innocent participant come within a hair's-breadth of killing someone or unleashing some cataclysmic event.

There is a concise clinical term for this kind of representation, but, not wanting to get sidetracked into a description of bovine excretory functions, I present the term's more delicate equivalent: nonsense. In this chapter, I will describe what hypnosis is, what it isn't, and what a person who has been hypnotized can and cannot be induced to do. (For a little bit about the history of hypnosis, see Appendix 2.)

What Hypnosis Isn't

I can't tell you how frustrating it is to me to see some old movie where the mad scientist uses hypnosis to turn his victim into a homicidal zombie. Sure, the movies are campy and entertaining, and I might even get a kick out of them if so many people didn't actually believe that such things were possible; but as a result, when hypnosis is recommended, otherwise intelligent people act as if you had just recommended that they submit to an exorcism or some gory voodoo ritual. Perhaps they fear that they will be brainwashed somehow, forced to submit their own personality to that of the practitioner. At the very least, too many people are concerned that they will be induced to do something humiliating, if not dangerous or illegal.

> A hypnotist can't make you do anything you don't really want to do. There's nothing spooky about it.
>
> **—Business Week**

Such fears, while long reinforced, are completely unfounded. For one thing, a hypnotized subject is never under any kind of "spell." Rather, he or she is completely conscious and aware of everything going on. Should the hypnotist suggest something — anything — that runs contrary to the subject's sensibilities, the subject would either ignore the suggestion or break off the session entirely, with no aftereffects. It is virtually impossible for anyone to impose anything upon a subject that is contrary to his or her will.

Another fear that may be present is the concern that, when experiencing hypnosis, a potential weaknesses in the subject's mental state might be exacerbated, with some previously undetected illness coming to the forefront. While this might be a tantalizing image upon which to build a horror movie, it is about as likely to occur as having the shadow on your bedroom wall at night actually turn into a terrifying monster and kill you.

Even some people who reject these absurd notions about hypnosis continue to hold to other myths that, while far less dramatic, are equally effective in preventing them from receiving the benefits available to them through hypnosis. For example, some people think that after a session or two, they will be completely changed into the kind of person they want to be. Upon discovering that they are still the same person they always were, they are likely to adopt an attitude of total skepticism about the process, often completely overlooking any positive effects they may have realized.

One more thing that hypnosis is not is that it is not a "miracle cure" or quick solution. As I stated, you cannot do anything you do not want to do, even when you are hypnotized. Thus, if you really do not want to lose weight (for whatever reason or reasons you may have), then hypnosis will have the same effect as the diet that you didn't follow or the exercise regimine that you didn't do. For hypnosis to work, you have to want it to work — and for that to happen, you have to want to lose those extra pounds.

What Hypnosis Really Is

Rather than being some form of subliminal coercion, hypnosis is a process whereby you allow yourself to do the things you really want to do and to put aside negative behaviors that you might have adopted during the course of your life. Perhaps the best way to define the process is to think of it as a cycle of permission which you grant to yourself.

Going back to the nightclub hypnotists, you've probably seen people brought on stage, hypnotized, then performing some silly act that they might normally find embarrassing. You'll note that nobody has ever been forced to do anything even remotely destructive or contrary to their moral code. They have just acted out the innate desire to be silly. We all acted on these desires as children, but were taught that the process of "growing up" precluded such behavior. The desire to be silly, however, lives on in each of us. We simply seek more "sophisticated" means of expressing it. When in the state of hypnosis, however, we have "permission" to allow that silliness to come through without the burden of our "grown-up" filters. So we prance about the stage like farm animals or stare at the audience as if we were looking at a crowd of naked people. Completely harmless, if potentially embarrassing.

Now if this idea of "permission" sounds ludicrous to you, think about this: Have you never caught yourself making bizarre faces in the mirror when you were alone in the bathroom, or singing (I should say, attempting to sing) like your favorite star, complete with theatrical gestures, when you were certain nobody could hear or see you? We both know that the answer is yes, even if the answer we speak aloud is no! In the privacy of your own solitude, you have given yourself the same permission you would when in the state of hypnosis.

Of course, hypnosis can be used for much more than simple entertainment, but the basic concept is the same. And if you recall, I described a cycle of permission. Here's how it works. Using hypnosis to access your genuine desires is, in and of itself, giving yourself permission to be yourself. The commitment to take steps to be what you want — whether that means being thinner, freer, a non-smoker, or whatever — is a clear statement to yourself. You are saying, "Yes, I allow myself to be thinner, free from addiction, less inhibited and shy, etc." Hypnosis, as a tool, simply reinforces that commitment and reconfirms the permission to do what you genuinely want to do. The two are intertwined, encouraging each other, and helping you progress toward the self you wish to be.

You have probably also seen news reports about how hypnosis can be used to reduce the pain a patient feels while undergoing some unpleasant medical procedure. A number of dentists utilize hypnosis as part or all of the anesthesia for performing even intense procedures such as root canals. You might think that the patient is in some deep trance, unable to feel or respond to pain. What actually takes place is that the patient is given permission to let go of his or her subjective interpretation of the physical sensations. We react to pain instinctively, out of a desire to avoid injury and survive. With the threat of trauma removed, we can respond more objectively to the pain itself, assigning to it no more significance than we would to a gentle brush across the arm or the smell of a rose. Without the emotional baggage we normally add to the physical sensation of pain, the pain becomes much less powerful. We simply observe it, as we would any other experience. Now, I'm not suggesting you run out and see just how much physical trauma you could withstand with the benefit of hypnosis. If I were, you would reject the suggestion, even if you were hypnotized. You would probably figure that my suggestion was physically impossible, and might even suggest that I attempt some physically impossible act in response!

While the use of hypnosis for anesthesia is something of an extreme example, it demonstrates both the

> My doctor told me to stop having intimate dinners for four. Unless there are three other people.
> —**Orson Welles**

potential and the limitations of hypnosis. Your own mind is capable of seemingly impossible feats when given permission to use more of its potential, yet you always retain your own unique will, which cannot be sublimated by another, no matter how skilled that person might be.

Most people don't realize that they have probably been "hypnotized" many times during the course of their lives. Now don't start getting paranoid! There is not some organized group of practitioners who go around putting people in trances when they aren't looking.[†] The truth is that each of us practices a form of self-hypnosis, virtually on a daily basis. For example, how many times have you spent considerable time driving along a familiar route, and upon reaching your destination, find that you can recall nothing of your drive? Being so well acquainted with the task at hand, you allowed your conscious mind to concentrate on other matters, while still handling the many tasks required to safely drive. You can easily recall the things you were thinking about as you drove, yet not the individual stops, starts, and turns of your journey. Only when some unfamiliar event occurred, such as the errant behavior of another driver or a change in road conditions, would your conscious focus return to your driving.

> In general, mankind, since the improvement of cookery, eats twice as much as nature requires.
>
> —**Benjamin Franklin**

To the other extreme, however, if we were to remain completely conscious of every decision we made while driving, it would be such a stress-filled activity

---

[†] Well, some would argue that the advertising industry regularly engages in this practice, but that's beyond the scope of this book.

that we would probably avoid driving at all costs. Remember when you were first learning to drive, and had to consciously focus on everything you did, such as how much pressure to apply to the accelerator and brake, and how far to turn the wheel to change lanes, while still judging what all the other drivers around you were doing? Although it might have been exciting at the time, the excitement of a new experience also contained the sheer terror of knowing you lacked the competence to be in the situation. Over time, as your sense of competence grew, the necessity of consciously observing every detail diminished, and you grew comfortable with the activity.

In much the same way, you can teach yourself to be confident — and competent — in other areas of your everyday life, allowing you to enjoy that life without becoming bogged down in details or ruled by petty emotions. Just as you became comfortable driving unconsciously as a result of sheer repetitiveness, you can consciously teach yourself how to achieve the same degree of comfort in other activities. The mechanism of your learning is the same.

In future chapters, I'll challenge you to become aware of the things that add stress to your life, and I will describe in detail the process for reducing that stress. While the focus of this book is weight control, I work with clients on many other issues as well, such as managing pain, reducing stress, improving grades, and optimizing athletic performance. But the effects of hypnosis can be far-reaching. Many of my weight-loss clients, for example, report that they are not only successful at reducing and maintaining their weight, but that they actually feel happier in other areas of their lives, as well. Such collateral effects are inevitable, since the things that make us unhappy — like being overweight — are rarely isolated from the other parts of our makeup, such as our overall self-image.

TOM **NICOLI**

My deepest desire is not just to help you get thin, but rather to help you put aside those things that rob your life of joy, whether they be pounds or fears. That said, let's proceed to the "nuts and bolts" and start building in you the permission to be happy. Once you have granted yourself that "permission", a sense of improved well being will follow.

How Hypnosis Actually Works

Now that we've gotten the myths surrounding hypnosis out of the way, the next step is to help you understand how hypnosis actually works and, more importantly, how you can make it can work for you. Though it is understandable and wise to approach a totally new activity with caution, I feel quite certain that once you become knowledgeable about how the process works, you will be comfortable enough to test it for yourself. And I have the feeling that once you've tried it, you will begin applying it to other aspects of your life besides weight loss. There is no real limit on the benefits you can realize from this simple endeavor once you get started.

Since very few readers will have a professional practitioner at their beck and call, I'm going to focus this discussion on the steps required to perform self-hypnosis. In this chapter, I will attempt to give you — without the added benefit of my melodiously soothing voice and calming music — the tools you will need to do it yourself. I will describe each step you will take before you take it, so that you not harbor lingering doubts that could prevent you from being successful.[†]

Whether you choose to undergo hypnotism with a qualified practitioner (see Appendix 4) or you decide to do it on your own, three factors must be in place in order for the

---

[†] In addition to my work with many individuals on a face-to-face basis, many thousands more have learned the process with the help of my series of audio CDs. On the CDs, I guide the listener step by step, using imagery and background music to facilitate their efforts. Please see the back of this book for more information.

process to work. These three factors are belief, desire and expectancy.

First you must believe hypnotism will work. It may seem as if I am asking you to take a leap of faith, but it isn't quite the same thing as having faith in a religious sense. To begin with, hypnotism has measurable and proven results. What it may require, however, is a suspension of disbelief, and for many people that's the hardest obstacle to overcome.

Second, you must have a genuine desire for hypnotism to work. This may seem self-evident, but the reality is that many people are torn between desiring change and fearing it. Not only must you unequivocally want to change, you must also truly want the process to work.

Finally, you must expect that hypnotism will work. This is not the same as merely believing; it is an absolute expectation that hypnotism will be effective in helping you make the changes you desire. You won't merely "try" to do it — after all, how many times have you "tried" in the past? No, this time you will do it!

If these three factors — belief, desire and expectancy — are in place, then you will be willing and open to suggestion. And you are ready to begin.

Getting Your Feet Wet...?

If being hypnotized doesn't mean being entranced and manipulated, then what does it mean? And how can you hypnotize yourself?

The keys to self-hypnosis are relaxation and imagination. The more relaxed you are, and the more vivid your imagined goal, the better your results will be. You will use pictures and/or words to communicate your goal to your subconscious. You need to make these words and images as powerful as possible, because the more convinced your subconscious mind is, the faster and greater the results.

As I had discussed earlier, hypnotism is best described as a cycle of permission to think, do, and be what we want. We are constantly being bombarded with experiences by the world we live in: sights, smells, tastes, sounds, and other physical sensations. On top of that, we tend to feed ourselves a pretty constant flow of thoughts and emotions inspired by experiences that are occurring right now, as well as memories of things that happened all the way back as far as we can remember. This constant flow of information can and does become pretty overwhelming, so it's not surprising that we may have a tough time finding the energy to change the things in our lives that we don't like.

Let me put it all in a more easily understood perspective. I have a friend who loves motorcycles. He already owns several, but is hungrily eyeing another one. Unfortunately, his garage is so full that he has absolutely no place to put the object of his current desire. He knows that before he can buy the new motorcycle, he has to clear out some space. So he goes into his garage and begins gathering up the "stuff" that no longer pleases him or serves a useful purpose. Just by organizing all that stuff and putting it in a more appropriate place, he soon clears enough space for his new toy.

> No matter how much pressure you feel at work, if you could find ways to relax for at least five minutes every hour, you'd be more productive.
> —**Dr. Joyce Brothers**

Similarly, in self-hypnosis, you will first need to "clear a space" in the clutter of your mind. This isn't as difficult as it may sound, because you're not "doing

60

anything" with the clutter. Instead, you will be consciously focusing upon the "clear" space you are looking for. To begin, you will need to be in a physical location that doesn't provide a lot of stimulation or place a lot of demands upon your conscious thoughts. It can be a quiet room in your home or office, or pretty much anywhere that you can escape telephones, television, radio, and interruptions by other people.[†]

Now that you've placed yourself in your "quiet zone", you can begin to redirect your thoughts to a single point, such as an imaginary spot on a wall. It is helpful (and, I believe, essential) to pay attention to your breathing when you begin, and structure your thoughts around it. As you take in a deep breath, you will imagine it nourishing you, filling you with healthful energy and peaceful feelings. As you gently release the breath, imagine that it carries with it all the things that bring stress to your life. You are breathing out the disagreement you had at work, the driver who cut you off, the noise that surrounds you every day. Inhaling deeply once again, you draw even deeper the nourishment you crave, and as you release the breath, you also release more of your stress. You will continue this cycle of nourishment and release, literally filling yourself with goodness, while eventually "sweeping out the corners" to remove any negative feelings you have.

As you continue consciously with this exercise, begin to notice how your body is responding. Focus on the muscles of your neck and shoulders, observing how they begin to loosen and relax. If they do not begin to grow more relaxed on their own, you should consciously relax them, one by one. As each area becomes more relaxed, move your focus down your body, relaxing each area in turn, then moving on to the next until you have reached and relaxed your feet and toes.

---

† Naturally, you would not want to attempt this while driving in your car. Beyond the difficulty of detaching yourself from the constant flow of stimulus, you would also be placing yourself and other drivers at risk by not focusing on your driving.

Now, observe how your entire body feels. You will notice that it doesn't feel all knotted up like it did before you started. You will continue breathing at a relaxed, yet conscious, rhythm, but you won't need to focus so closely upon that rhythm. After only a few minutes of doing this, you will discover that your mind, as well as your body, will feel much more relaxed. It is at this point that your mind is most open and receptive to conscious, positive input. Right now, your focus has moved beyond the little details that usually occupy you, to drift into the realm of your unconscious. Thoughts and emotions become less significant. Believe it or not, you are hypnotized! You are not entranced or impeded in any way, but rather, capable of functioning on an objective, more spiritual level. The sense of peacefulness you experience will be quite refreshing, yet will not cloud your perception of anything going on in your daily life.

I take it that what all men are really after is some form or perhaps only some formula of peace.

—Joseph Conrad

By merely practicing this simple exercise on a regular basis, you will realize substantial benefits. Your blood pressure will probably be lowered, and your sense of well being will be enhanced. This practice actually has its origins in the meditation rituals of many of the world's religions, and is virtually identical to meditation techniques that are growing continually more popular.[†]

It is in this state that you will be more able to listen to your genuine needs, the hungers you feel beyond

62

† Although there are a few religions that claim such practices to be "sinful" or somehow destructive, I prefer an approach that describes it like this: if prayer is talking to God, meditation (and by extension, hypnotism) is listening to God. Judging by some of the things we do to ourselves during our day-to-day "conscious" lives, we could all benefit from getting quiet and just listening now and then!

expectations and external influences. Old habits will seem less ingrained. You will more objectively observe the things you have done that held you back from being the person you want to be. It is in this space of peaceful, focused "drifting" that you will give yourself the permission to be better, happier, and healthier.

Your mind will be more rational, less confused by the "chatter" of negative thoughts. You will begin to see that many of the things that you deemed important are really distractions, whose importance has been established by others (or even yourself), and blindly accepted as being real. It is by letting go of these distractions that you can begin to build upon your genuine needs and desires, and to experience — perhaps for the first time — what it is to be truly free.

I realize that the activity I have described will seem quite unfamiliar to many people. After all, we spend virtually every waking moment in silent discussion with ourselves, explaining, justifying, and even rationalizing our thoughts, behaviors, and the circumstances of our lives. To step beyond the pattern of dialog that has been so prevalent in your life can seem almost impossible, especially when the dialog itself seems determined to retain its predominance. You may even tell yourself that it just won't work for you, or that you are one of those people who just can't be hypnotized.

> There is no need to go to India or anywhere else to find peace. You will find that deep place of silence right in your room, your garden or even your bathtub.
> **—Elisabeth Kubler-Ross**

Such arguments are just part of that very dialog that we're trying to move beyond. See how effective it is at

63

surviving? In truth, this process will work for anyone who wants it to work and is willing and open to trying. Remember those three factors: belief, desire and expectancy!

And then remember that fourth factor: permission. As I've said before, by giving yourself permission to try something different to improve your life, you will be accessing the mechanism of permission to go beyond the limitations you have placed upon yourself. It's a wonderful, powerful cycle that has worked for many thousands of people. Isn't it time to make it work for you?

The exercise above was merely to give you a taste of self-hypnosis. If you feel it didn't "work", then don't worry. In future chapters I will go into more detail about the actual process. You may become very adept at doing it yourself just by reading this book. Or you may choose to use a CD or tape, or even consult with a qualified practitioner. In any case, I think it is important that we first take a little more time to discuss the three critical factors of belief, desire, and expectancy. While it seems that some "new" belief system is popping up every day, demanding that its adherents blindly accept alien concepts as truth, there is no such demand where the practice of hypnotism is concerned. I have no patience with airy-fairy rituals that are too "sophisticated" for us earthlings to comprehend. Instead, we will talk about how you can use your innate intelligence and good common sense to give yourself the permission to overcome the factors that have hindered your journey to happiness for so long. And then we will go more deeply into the "how-to's" of self-hypnosis. After that, we'll discuss the specific tasks you will undertake in your efforts to manage your weight. The ultimate goal you will reach if you follow along will be not only weight loss, but a sense of happiness and general well-being. And what more could you ask from any system or technique?

Belief, Desire, and Expectancy

In the previous section, I briefly discussed the three factors essential to your success with using hypnotism: **belief**, **desire**, and **expectancy**. Although these might seem to be pretty straightforward, they typically represent the most difficult obstacles to overcome, as we tend to overlook the unconscious elements that are such powerful influences on our thinking. In this section, I will attempt to clarify what each represents, and how you can move beyond the obstacles that so many people face.

Belief

Naturally, before you can even begin to use a process such as hypnotism, you must believe that it actually works. And being an intelligent person[†], you will need some degree of proof. While each of us might take a "leap of faith" from time to time, our common sense and survival instincts prevent us from taking that leap completely blind.

> Creative power is that receptive attitude of expectancy which makes a mold into which the plastic and as yet undifferentiated substance can flow and take the desired form.—**Thomas Troward**

The most direct route to helping you believe that hypnosis is real — and that you can be hypnotized — would be to sit down with you, face to face for an hour and demonstrate the procedure. Inasmuch as most people who read this book will probably never come to my office or one of my workshops, such a solution is impractical. Another option would be to listen to self-hypno-

---

† You are obviously an intelligent person because you exercised the good judgment to read this book!

sis CDs offered by a reputable practitioner. For those of you who want instant gratification, there are literally hundreds of case studies and articles containing unsolicited feedback, and these are available either at the public library or online. Try going online and typing the words 'hypnosis' and 'effective' in your favorite search engine. You'll find a long list of references, which I won't even attempt to list here.

Of course, the results of your search would be purely intellectual, and might still fail to overcome your healthy skepticism. But if you add the empirical data supporting the validity of hypnosis to your own experiences described in earlier (remember where I described the experience of driving somewhere, yet being unable to recall the details of the trip?), you may very well discover that your skepticism begins to diminish. Full-fledged belief in the potential of hypnotism may take a little longer, but you'll get there.

Desire

If you're like most people, the desire part is easy — at least on the surface. We all want to find that magic process, pill, or diet that takes us from where we are to where we want to be. It would seem, then, that the desire would have been in place before you ever picked up this book. But if you look at that desire honestly, it turns out that your yearning is for the result you seek, rather than for the success of a specific means to your desired end. The desire is actually for a thinner you, rather than for hypnotism to work for you. So how can you translate the desire for thinness into a desire for hypnotism to get you there? It's a simple process of elimination.

Unless you awakened this morning and decided for the first time that you wanted to lose weight, you've probably tried a number of methods already. Every magazine at the supermarket checkout proclaims in big, bold letters that it holds the latest, most effective "magic bullet" to help you lose weight. Even though a significant part of my practice is devoted to weight control, I don't even try to keep track of all the "miracle" programs that come out every month. After all, if any of them worked, the number of obese people in the supermarket — and the world — would begin to diminish, given the millions of people who read the magazines and try out the miracle of the month.

You might have done your time as a "gym rat", spending countless hours on very sophisticated machines. You might also have taken all the over-the-counter weight loss products you could buy, only to find yourself jittery and sleepless, but still overweight. The list could go on a lot longer, but you get the point. It has been said that it is foolish — even crazy — to try the same things over and over while expecting a different result. When you consider that all the magic remedies have been available in various forms for many years, yet we as a species are growing more obese every day, it seems logical to assume that the magical remedies of the hour just aren't working. And you want something that works, right?

If you can look beyond the prejudice we've already discussed, and look honestly at all the methods that you've used unsuccessfully to lose weight, I think you'll find that hypnosis starts looking pretty good, and that you may begin to desire for it to be effective for you. So much for the second hurdle!

Expectancy

At this point, you are probably well on your way to clearing the third hurdle: the expectation that hypnosis will work for you. It has been my experience that, even though you may still harbor some doubts at this point, by going forward with even a hesitant belief, coupled with a genuine desire to succeed, you will quickly discover that hypnotism is not only real, but highly effective and quite pleasant. By experiencing only the subtlest form of hypnosis, you will find yourself much more relaxed and freed from much of the stress that seemed to hang over you. With each subsequent session, you will find yourself growing more comfortable with hypnosis. The fears and doubts you had early on will fade away, and your expectation of positive experiences and results will continue to grow. Like anything else, the more you do it, the better you will get at it, and the easier and more pleasant the experience will become.

However, don't get discouraged if everything doesn't fall immediately into place. It might take a few tries before you begin to feel that you've "got it." Keep in mind that you've spent a lot of years developing the mindset and habits that stand in the way of complete success in your weight loss efforts. It might take a few weeks to put aside any misconceptions or misgivings you may have, but I feel confident you will be able to do it, as have thousands of people with whom I've worked.

In the next chapter, I'll discuss in greater detail the actual process of hypnotizing yourself, and give you directions as to how you can apply your newly acquired skills to the specific task of losing and managing your weight.

Thin **Thoughts**

Hypnosis is a process whereby you allow yourself to do the things you really want to do and to put aside negative behaviors that you might have adopted during the course of your life.

Hypnosis, as a tool, simply reinforces that commitment and reconfirms the permission to do what you genuinely want to do.

The keys to self-hypnosis are relaxation and imagination.

By giving yourself permission to try something different to improve your life, you will be accessing the mechanism of permission to go beyond the limitations you have placed upon yourself.

The mirror of self-reflection is clouded with excuses and reasons and is cleared with truth and honesty.

— **Tom Nicoli**

CHAPTER 6 THINKING THIN

8 Steps to Self Hypnosis

In the last chapter, I gave a brief overview of the process of hypnotizing yourself. This time, I want to describe in detail the steps you'll take to experience self-hypnosis, with specific attention devoted to helping you develop a healthier way of looking at and living your life. The most important thing for you to remember is that nothing I describe will be alien to you. Everything you do will be absolutely natural; you will simply be responding to the actual needs of your body and spirit, rather than the artificial demands we so frequently place upon ourselves.

8 Steps to Self-hypnosis

Step 1. Location, location, location

It is important that you are in a physical location that is conducive to getting relaxed, one where you won't have a bunch of interruptions to distract you. You will want to find a place that is reasonably quiet, and where (ideally) nobody knows how to reach you. So close out your e-mail program, turn off your cell phone, the TV, radio, and any other source of outside stimulus that might be prattling in the background. You will want about twenty or thirty minutes of peaceful solitude, so choose a place where you can reasonably expect to stay that long without being disturbed. If you have a home office, that is ideal as you can close the door and lock the world out. As long as you have a quiet place in your home where you can be by yourself, you'll be fine.

Step 2. It's your song…choose lyrics and images carefully.

Imagine that you are assigned the task of writing a simple song about yourself as you would like to be. If your goal is to lose weight, first imagine yourself as being thin and healthy. Think of how proud you are of your healthy, focused self. Look closely at the image in the mirror of your mind, noticing all the details. See the bright smile that looks back at you, the toned, powerful legs that carry you, and the firm, lithe body that is yours. Then choose simple words and phrases that describe that image and hold those words and phrases in your mind. They will serve as reminders of the rewards that you will be giving yourself. Here are a few examples, but feel free to come up with your own:

Flat tummy

Firm thighs

Toned arms

Strong

Supple

Proud

Bright eyes

You get the picture. Describe someone you would want to know, but keep in mind that these words accurately describe you as you were meant to be.

Once you have your mental list made up, begin to expand it to include the things that will help you achieve your goals, but have so far proven difficult to embrace. For example, you might include phrases such as these:

Eat light

Eat healthy

Have abundant energy

Exercise daily

Feed the machine

Remember that these key words and phrases are powerful beacons for the path you are embarking upon, so you won't want to imagine them written in small letters on a page. Instead, let them be bold neon lights that illuminate the sky, as is befitting their power and majesty.

Step 3. Are you sitting comfortably?

Actually, that's the name of an old song by the Moody Blues, and I think they had the right idea. Throughout the ages, different meditation practices have demanded that the student adopt complicated (and often, uncomfortable) postures in order to achieve a meditative state. While self-hypnosis is closely akin to meditation, it is wholly unnecessary — even counterproductive — to devote your energy to a physical position or posture that is alien to you.

Instead, you will want to either sit comfortably (yes...in a chair is fine, if that's what is most comfortable to you) or lie down. If you are sitting, keep both feet flat on the ground and your hands lying flat in your lap, loose and comfortable. If you're lying down, let your legs lie straight, with your feet about eighteen inches apart, toes pointing slightly outward, completely relaxed. Your hands should fall flat by your sides, completely relaxed.

If it seems strange to focus so intently upon your physical positioning, you should remember that the ultimate goal of your self-hypnosis is to achieve a state of comfortable balance in your life, so it only makes sense that you begin your journey in a position of comfortable balance. For example, even if you find it comfortable to sit with your legs crossed, in such a position, some of your muscles would be relaxed, while others are stretched taut. Furthermore, sitting in that position for an extended period of time can impair the circulation in your legs and damage sensitive veins. On the other hand, by adopting a position such as I have described in the previous paragraph, your body will be working in synch with your mental images toward a common goal.

Step 4. Breathe!

Begin by taking a few deep breaths, drawing deeply in through your nose, filling your diaphragm so that your belly rises, rather than your chest. You do not need to inhale so deeply that it feels unnatural or strained, just enough that you have the sensation of being filled. Hold each breath for about five seconds, then release it gently through your mouth. As you draw each breath into your body, imagine pure, clean oxygen rushing into your lungs. As you hold each breath, imagine your body being deeply nourished. Then, as you release each breath, see yourself gently releasing all the toxins that you have harbored in your body. All the anxiety, tension, stress, anger, and sadness that have filled you are released in the breath. They are not cast out in anger, but released as something you no longer need.

After these deep breaths, allow your breathing to return to its own natural rhythm. There is no need to force anything, as your breath knows its proper way. But in each breath, you continue to breathe in nourishment and nurturing, while releasing those things that do not serve you.

Step 5. Awash in calm

As you continue following and observing the natural rhythm of your breathing, you will notice that you are becoming more and more relaxed and calm. Begin to focus that calmness on specific parts of your body, starting at the top of your head and working down. Though I would assume that you rarely give the muscles in your scalp and face much thought, observe how pleasant is the sensation when those muscles begin to relax. Allow your jaw muscles to go slack, and you will notice how tense they typically are. If you're like me, you probably tend to carry a lot of tension in the muscles of your neck. As you breathe away your tension, feel the cords in your neck begin to grow soft and supple.

Now continue this process all the way down your body, through all the muscle groups, until you reach the tips of your toes. You will always be breathing away the tension and stress, while taking in the pure nourishment your body requires. As you continue, you will notice that your breathing becomes more calm, as well. Its pace slows somewhat, falling into its own languid rhythm, further encouraging the sense of calm and the relaxed state of your entire body.

> You are never too old to set another goal or to dream a new dream.
>
> **—C.S. Lewis**

Step 6. Stepping deeper

As you continue to become more relaxed, imagine yourself at the top of a stairway or on an elevator. There

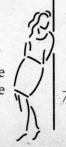

75

are ten steps or floors below you, and you begin to slowly descend. At each step or floor, repeat to yourself, "Deeper." When you reach the bottom, tell yourself, "I am there." You are now in a state of deep hypnosis.

You are still in your silent place, and more "in control" than before you began. It is in this place that you are best equipped to deal with those things that have compromised your physical well being and robbed you of joy, for all that exists in this place is the truth of who you are, what you feel, and what you need.

Step 7. Focusing on your goals

Remember the images and phrases I discussed in Step 2? It is at this point that you will actually begin putting them to use. While you are in the deepest, most relaxed state of hypnosis, you will be most receptive to suggestions, and you will be able to build a lasting picture in your subconscious mind. That's why it's so important that you choose the most powerful words and images possible. As you picture yourself thinner, healthier, and happier, you won't be struggling with the negative "chatter" that you have learned over the course of your lifetime.

If you repeatedly draw upon those images of what you hope to become, you will eventually replace the old, negative images with the newer, positive ones, and will begin to actually see yourself in a better light.

At this point, even the skepticism you might have harbored about the whole process will be overpowered by a sense of optimism, borne of truth that is freed from the disappointments you have experienced in the past.

Continue repeating your key phrases and recalling those positive images for as long as you are comfortable doing so, or until you have used up all the time you have allotted to the exercise. Then, we go to the eighth and final step.

Step 8. Emergence!

When you are finished with your imaging, you will begin to count yourself out of your sacred place. Imagine riding that same elevator back up, beginning on level ten and counting backwards to one. As you rise to each successive level, acknowledge a new and vibrant energy coursing through your being. Affirm the feeling with phrases at each step, such as:

I am more energized than I have ever felt!

I feel better than I have ever felt!

I feel physically stronger than I have ever felt!

My spirit feels stronger than ever before!

I am more alert than ever before!

I can do anything I want to do!

When you get back to level one, think, "I am now alert, and feel wonderful in every way!"

It is not the mountain we conquer but ourselves.
—**Edmund Hillary**

Set aside a time to do this exercise at least once (but preferably twice) every day, and keep it up for at least three weeks in a row. You will notice real changes for the better in yourself, even in this short amount of time. You will also find that, as you continue, it will be easier and easier for you to achieve a deep, relaxed state, and that it will take you less time to get there. The best part is that, unlike so many other efforts to change yourself, the changes you will realize through self-hypnosis will be permanent.

As you can see, there is no real mystery involved in hypnotism, and once you have tried the exercise, I feel certain that any uneasiness you might once have felt will disappear. Furthermore, you will probably find yourself anxiously looking forward to your next session, eager to once again feel that sense of calm and certainty that hypnotism brings. While you might have initially thought that it would be difficult to commit to a half-hour, twice a day, you will quickly discover that it is no more a burden than doing anything else you truly enjoy.

In the next chapter, I will discuss ways to fine-tune your self-hypnosis to specifically address your goals of weight reduction and improvement of your overall physical well being. Beyond that, your imagination is the only limit upon the areas of your life where hypnotism can offer improvement.

Thin **Thoughts**

I am more energized than I have ever felt!

I feel better than I have ever felt!

I feel physically stronger than I have ever felt!

My spirit feels stronger than ever before!

I am more alert than ever before!

I can do anything I want to do!

The last time I *tried* was another time I didn't *do*.

— **Tom Nicoli**

CHAPTER 7

THINKING THIN

Applying Hypnotism to Weight Loss

In the previous chapter, I took you step by step through the process of self-hypnosis. If you've practiced even a few times, you have probably discovered that you felt more relaxed, and that the things that made your life stressful have become less powerful. This is a great start! The next step will be to learn how to make focused, conscious suggestions, with weight loss and control being the primary objective. Beyond merely losing weight, however, you will begin to notice yourself gravitating toward feelings and behaviors that improve your overall physical, intellectual, and emotional well being.

The suggestions we will focus upon will not feel strange to you, and will not be contrary to any beliefs you may hold. On the contrary, they will feel completely natural. This is because nature has created a state of inherent balance in all things, including human behavior. Through the course of our lives, we tend to take ourselves out of that state of balance. It's not a conscious act but a subconscious one, making it all the more powerful and difficult to reverse. We fall out of balance because of misleading, incorrect information we are repeatedly given. By implanting the correct information while in the highly receptive state of hypnosis, we are able to direct our attitudes and behaviors at the same subconscious level where we have received all the misleading information that has held us down. This is what I mean by "giving yourself permission" to restore the balance in your life. As you become more aware of the essential truth that is borne of that balance, every part of you will accept the change in your outlook.

Okay, so how do you use the powerful tool of hypnotism to manage your weight? Any good weight loss or weight management program incorporates healthy eating habits and proper exercise. So let's start with eating.

To begin with, you need to acknowledge that your appetite is a product of your inherent survival instinct. In truth, the act of eating isn't just an optional behavior — it is a responsibility. Giving your body what it needs to survive and prosper is your primary job. Before you were ever seduced by thousands of hours of commercials, cajoled by parents to eat a certain way, prodded by peers to partake of certain things, or programmed by the workplace to eat at certain times, you were guided by a simple motivation: you ate when you were hungry, you ate until you were satisfied, and when you were no longer hungry, you stopped eating. Sounds simple, doesn't it? It was, and still is (or rather, it should be!).

> To avoid sickness eat less; to prolong life worry less.
> —**Chu Hui Weng**

Unfortunately, as we grew older, we were no longer afforded the luxury of a constantly available breast or bottle, and our eating habits began moving from the realm of survival to one of social interaction. Even in kindergarten, we ate cookies and milk at a certain time each day, and were informed that the cookies were more delectable than apples and carrots and the like. Just as our subconscious learned to comply with the norms and schedules of others, our bodies also learned to adapt.

As we told our bodies to wait until it was "time" to eat, they reacted by reverting to their most fundamental survival techniques. Even though your body needed nourishment at ten in the morning, for instance, you made it wait until lunchtime. Imagine your body's reaction: "Here we go again...famine time. I'd better start storing nutrients so that I can survive until I get my next meal, whenever that may be." And how does your body store nutrients? By depositing them in fat cells, rather than allowing them to be used to generate energy. So the next time you ate, instead of the food going to muscle tissue to make you healthier, it went to fat tissue.

As discussed earlier in this book, that is why diets based upon withholding food don't really work, and even make you get fatter in the long run. To effectively lose and manage your weight, you will need to stop giving your body bad information that tricks it into getting fatter. Give it good information, and you'll soon find that supplying your body's needs will no longer be "discipline" — it will be second nature.

> To eat is a necessity, but to eat intelligently is an art.
> —**La Rochefoucauld**

Good Information Equals Good Health

Here is a significant point that I want to emphasize. It's imperative that you realize this. When you eat the proper, small amounts of healthy food to satisfy your

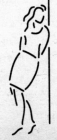

Some Truly Thin Thoughts...

I eat when I am hungry. At the first sign of hunger, I will eat a few bites of food.

I stop eating when I am full. I won't eat with any goal in mind beyond that of feeling satisfied. I don't need to clean my plate or take a second helping to make the chef feel appreciated.

I eat light. I choose to eat sufficient food to make me feel good, rather than enough to make me feel full.

I am satisfied. See "I eat light."

I've had enough. Self-explanatory...The trick for many of us is determining when enough is enough!

I eat healthy. I choose foods that are healthful and nourishing. I avoid heavy foods, greasy foods, and foods that are hard to digest.

Less fat is best. The more fat on my plate, the more that will settle in my butt, waist, thighs...you get the point.

Baked is beautiful. Think fish and chicken, though — not cakes and pies!

Broiled is sublime.

Nothing fried.[†]

I am energized. My food makes me feel alive, not sleepy or sluggish.

Eat fresh. I relish all the nutrients in foods, rather than cooking them to death.

I feel the life in the foods I eat. Fresh vegetables, fruits, and nuts.

I need less meat. While a strict vegetarian diet isn't necessary for good health, neither is eating the equivalent of an entire cow every year!

My body is water. I will drink water to replenish it.

84

† No offense to my Southern friends, many of whom claim that "if it ain't fried, it ain't food."

physical hunger, you will — and actually do need to — eat more often. When you eat a small amount of healthy food, your metabolism adjusts to the message that there will always be enough food when needed, and it burns fat, rather than storing it against future lack. Isn't it nice to know that you can eat more often and reduce fat more quickly at the same time?

Before you even opened your eyes at birth, your body was fully capable of deciding when it was time to eat, how much to eat, and even what to eat. But over time, you thought you had gotten smarter than your body. You were wrong! On the previous page, I give you words and phrases (some truly thin thoughts!) that you can use during your self-hypnosis sessions to overcome the misinformation that has hampered your process for so long.

You will want to expand upon this list, using simple phrases that are especially descriptive to you. The important thing in choosing your key words and phrases is that they are focused on helping you remember what it is like to eat naturally, as your body needs, rather than artificially, as most of us have done for the better part of our lives.

Beyond the lists, learn to listen to what your body tells you when you eat or drink. How do different foods and beverages make you feel? Make a list, like the one below, of words that describe how you feel physically after eating a meal. Recall how you felt after eating, and see whether the words in list A or list B better describe that feeling.

List A	List B
Stuffed	Energized
Lazy	Excited
Full	Satisfied
Sleepy	Refreshed

Bloated	Relaxed
Miserable	Comfortable
Heavy	Light
Hot	Cool

Remember a time when you ate a big Porterhouse steak, baked potato (with all the trimmings, of course), bread and butter, and followed it with a decadently rich dessert? Which of the above lists best describes the way you felt? Now recall a hot summer day, when you felt thirsty. If you drank a carbonated beverage, you probably enjoyed its sweetness, and the cold liquid felt good going down, but how did you feel afterward? If you're like most people, you probably still felt thirsty. Yet, if you recall another occasion, when you drank a glass of cold water or juice, you probably felt refreshed and energized. Observe which list best describes your feelings.

The words in List B describe a healthier physical state, while those in List A describe a state that is not very consistent with health. Since it has long been proven that the healthiest specimens of any species are the ones that survive and flourish, doesn't it make sense to seek out things that make you feel healthier, and therefore, more prepared to survive? Granted, the commercials we see are pretty effective at convincing us that we want more fatty foods, and few of us (especially kids) are immune to the allure of advertisements for burgers and soft drinks. But the folks who pay for those commercials are interested in the health of their companies' stocks, not in the physical health of their customers. It is up to you to "advertise" to your unconscious mind the kinds of foods that will best serve your body.

If you still need to be convinced, or just want some extra "inspiration" for healthier eating, rent the movie **Super Size Me**, a documentary by Morgan Spurlock.[†] This is the somewhat harrowing tale of how a healthy man in his mid-thir-

---

† Warning: Do not watch this movie while you are eating, but you might think about it the next time you feel tempted to order that jumbo bag of fries.

ties became an overweight sluggard with potentially serious health problems — after only thirty days of dining on nothing but items from a famous fast-food chain. The documentary also presents some pretty frightening statistics about how the "typical American diet" is wreaking havoc on our collective health and waistlines.

The point I want you to remember is that changing your diet is not about deprivation, just retraining. By following the steps I provide, you will actually feel happier eating healthy foods in healthy quantities. And in addition to feeling healthier and happier, you will have a higher degree of self respect and pride, because you will know that you are truly creating a better you.

In the next chapter, we will discuss ways to use self-hypnosis to teach yourself the joy of exercise. Don't worry! I have no interest in turning you into an obsessive gym rat or one of those people who have to run three miles every day in order to feel okay. Now that you understand hypnotism more completely, you know that I couldn't do it, even if I wanted to.

The philosophy of one century is the common sense of the next.

— **Henry Ward Beecher**

CHAPTER 8

Make Exercise Exciting

In the previous chapter, we discussed some methods of delivering suggestions to your subconscious mind that would encourage you to eat healthier foods, at the right times, in the right quantities, and for the right reasons. With very little practice, you will find yourself following a diet that is much better for what your body really needs. And that's a great start.

However, in order to really get yourself on track to a healthy lifestyle, you will need to keep your body actively burning up the foods you do eat. Even if you're eating only healthy, nutritious foods, you will not lose much weight — and could even continue to gain — if you don't maintain an activity level sufficient to use up nutrients, rather than just storing them. That's where exercise comes in.[†]

Now, I realize that, for many people, exercise is a concept that rates right up there with a root canal on the fun scale. Perhaps you tell yourself that since you work hard all day it's just too inconvenient to think about undertaking an exer-

---

† Although exercise is essential to physical and emotional well being, it is important that you not overwhelm yourself with an exercise routine that is beyond your capacity. Before beginning any exercise regimen, you should get a checkup from a health care provider who is aware of your intentions, particularly if you are of the Baby Boomer generation or older. You should set the pace of your exercise program to your own abilities and aspirations, rather than some external goal. That way, your efforts will result in success rather than frustration, and you won't risk harm to your physical health by attempting a routine that isn't right for you. You aren't looking to be a running back, just a better you.

cise program. After all, you only have so much energy, right? When you finish your workday, all you want to do is curl up with a good meal and a video and unwind. Besides, if you're working that hard, you might figure you are getting all the exercise you need.

That's understandable, if misguided. Just as most people have been "taught" to eat poorly, they have also been taught that the work they do during the day is all they are capable of and that it provides them with their daily requirement of exercise. The bottom line is that they have been taught wrong — and their bodies are paying the price.

By now, you know that it is impossible to use hypnotism to convince yourself that something distasteful or unpleasant is really fun, so we won't even try. What we will attempt to do is to help you unlearn your erroneous belief that exercise is a chore. And the first step will be to help you remember a time in your life when you didn't see it that way.

It is exercise alone that supports the spirits, and keeps the mind in vigor.

—**Cicero**

If you look back to your childhood, you can recall a time when you ran, jumped, skipped, swam, and shouted at the top of your lungs, just for the pure joy of the act. You certainly weren't doing so because you were committed to your health; you acted out of a sense of pure fun. So what happened to you that took the fun away?

For many, your fun was inevitably cut short by the need to attend to some responsibility, like schoolwork or cleaning up your room. Even your instinctive practice of what you now know to be self-hypnosis or meditation was probably discouraged by the oft-repeated admonishment to "stop daydreaming and do something."

Your biggest challenge, then, is to recall and rekindle the sense of joy you had many years ago, and to make that joy real to you once again.

Just as you did in the chapter on using self-hypnosis to achieve weight loss, you will begin by gathering helpful images of how you really want to be and feel, then consolidating those images into a list of key words and phrases to use while in hypnosis. Since it may have been a long time since you felt the absolute joy of playing, I will try to help you along with some images that work for me. If one or more of these images touches the right nerve for you, let yourself build upon it until it is your own.

All right...let's begin.

It's a beautiful spring day. A Saturday. The temperature is cool, but not cold at all. There are cartoons playing on television, and you watched them while you ate your breakfast, but as soon as the last corner of toast was washed down with the last sip of juice, you felt something beckoning you outside. The call was so strong that you might have left your dishes right there on the table. Mom will probably scold you for not clearing them away, but her admonishment is a future thing, and doesn't really exist for you. All that matters is outside. Running out the door into the yard, you feel the rush of cool air on your face. It feels and smells like it's never been breathed before, created in this moment for your pleasure alone.

The doctor of the future will give no medicine, but instead will interest his patients in the care of the human frame, in diet, and in the cause and prevention of disease.—**Thomas Edison**

91

It isn't enough to just feel the breeze. You must run head-long into it, with no particular destination in mind other than the immediate sensation of coolness. You run faster, as if to satisfy a hunger for the breeze that will not be sated, but grows ever stronger as it is fed. As you keep running, you imagine yourself on the bridge of a schooner, rushing toward a horizon you cannot see. Or perhaps you imagine what it must feel like to fly like a bird, with no contact with the world except the wind itself. And you fly higher. Faster. Joy is no longer a word to you, or even an idea you can wrap your mind around. It is the feeling of the wind on your face, of your legs pumping harder and faster. After a few minutes that feel like the sum total of your existence, you begin to slow a bit. Your legs feel a little tired, but they feel so good, so alive. Your breathing is deeper and faster; your body hungry for its own taste of the coolness that brought you outside. And for a mo-ment after you stop, you feel a flush of heat across your face until the breeze begins to whisper away the sweat.

Now hold that moment. Savor the sensations. And re-member the smile that beamed from your face for no reason other than its own existence. In those moments, your body was speaking absolute truth to you. It liked the way it felt when you used it. This was not a chore, not a responsibility. This was fun. Perhaps sometime in the far future, as a grown-up, you might think you looked silly, sprinting to nowhere wearing a grin that stretched from your toes to the sky. But there is nobody observing you now, and if they are, they simply don't exist in your universe. In this universe, all that exists is you, your body fully engaged in song and dance with the greater world.

Now, I want you to imagine yourself running in your present body, in your present state of mind. The sensation is dramatically different, isn't it? Nowadays, if you run at all, it is probably a means to an end, rather than an end in itself. Perhaps you're sprinting down an airport terminal, afraid you'll miss the final boarding call. Or you might be chasing your dog, who dashed beneath your legs and out the door to taste freedom, if only for a little while. Or maybe you are jogging down the running trail in the park, determined to beat your best time around the circuit. Good for the heart, you know. And when it's over, you will reward yourself with a cappuccino and croissant. All that is missing is the joy you felt that fine spring day, so long ago. It has been replaced by objectives.

If you are going to turn exercise from a chore into a pleasure, the first step will be to change those objectives. Notice that I am not asking you to do away entirely with objectives, but rather to put aside the artificial priorities you have been taught and replace them with the more organic priorities that your body sets when it is allowed. I don't expect you to jump up and run willy-nilly out your kitchen door (though it might serve to break up your neighbors' boredom); however, you can certainly begin to listen to your body a bit more closely and respond to what it needs when freed of the "priorities" you have artificially imposed upon it. And don't worry...you needn't completely abandon your hard-earned adulthood in the process!

The goal in life is living in agreement with nature.

—**Zeno**

As a matter of fact, you will find that actually listening to what your body really needs will be the most mature thing you can do. Even though you will be relearning the process of having pure, unadulterated fun, you will be reassured by the knowledge that your actions are both logical and productive.

TOM **NICOLI**

As a kid, you worked hard at your fun, probably even harder than you do to meet your grownup responsibilities. The difference is that your focus then was completely upon the joy of the sensations you experienced. Where you got sidetracked was in accepting the erroneous notion that those wonderful sensations were incompatible with adult life.

Just think about it: When you were a child, you did those things that made your body and your spirit feel good. Your actions felt good because they fulfilled some genuine need, even though you didn't understand the need at the time. The needs are still there, even though you might not understand them now.

To really understand your body's need for exercise, try thinking about it as a complex organic machine (which it is, after all). Like any machine, your body needs to be used in order to maintain its efficiency. Leave your car in the garage for six months without driving it, and you'll get an idea of what happens to your body when it is deprived of exercise for an extended period of time. If you're lucky, you'll only need a jump to get the thing started. If you're not so lucky, parts inside will have grown so accustomed to their positioning that they simply won't move. In a car, we refer to that in terms like rust or corrosion. In our bodies, we use terms like atrophy. The bottom line is that if you want either machine to perform, you need to use it as it was intended on a regular basis in order to keep it limber. At the very worst, if something is going wrong, you'll get some indication of the problem before it ceases to

> People say that losing weight is no walk in the park. When I hear that I think, yeah, that's the problem.
> —**Chris Adams**

94

Key Phrases for Exercise...

I love how my body feels when I exercise.

Being fit is my birthright.

Active = joyous

My body is a thoroughbred machine.

My body loves to exert itself.

Running for joy.

A healthy glow.

I enjoy exercise.

I respect my body.

I reap rewards from physical activity.

I am stronger and healthier as I exercise.

My body requires exercise and I enjoy it.

I remove limitations in my life.

Growing fitter every day.

Burning away the sludge that slows me down.

I am growing stronger and more fit every day.

I feel more alive than I did yesterday.

I will look and feel even better tomorrow.

I am proud of how I look and feel.

function completely. And at the very best, the well-used machine will adapt to regular use by becoming more efficient over time. The fact that using the machine can be a lot of fun — while actually having some productive benefit — should appeal to even the most diehard grownup in you.

Toward that end, I have developed a short list of key words and phrases that have proven useful in hypnosis sessions. (You'll find that list on the next page.) You will, of course, want to modify the list, adding phrases that have particular meaning for you. The only "rules" are that you keep the images simple and focused upon those phrases that are geared toward meeting your body's real needs, while still being comprehensible to an inherently fun-challenged adult mind. Once you get started, you'll find that it's not that difficult, and you really enjoy the process. And once you apply the images to your self-hypnosis, you'll discover that you actually enjoy exercise, maybe even as much as you did so many years ago.

The last item on the list represents a springboard to even higher levels of physical and mental well being. Those of us who have experienced a sluggish, sedentary lifestyle might tell ourselves we don't even think about doing things differently. The truth is that by making such a statement to yourself, you are not merely misleading your conscious mind, you are feeding into a type of depression that literally robs you of joy. Even if you deny thinking about your own level of physical fitness, you may find that thoughts, daydreams, and nighttime dreams will repeatedly intrude, reminding you, for example, of how wonderful it feels to run, jump, or even fly. This is your subconscious mind trying to nudge you — to remind you — of what you really need. I have a friend with emphysema who says he frequently dreams about the days in his youth when he used to run and run, never getting tired or winded. He had these dreams (and daydreams) for years before he finally quit smoking cigarettes and started riding his bicycle (which he had always loved doing). It took him a while to restore his body to the point where he didn't tire immediately, but he felt so good about himself that he eventually found he was seeking out reasons to exercise, rather than excuses to avoid it. His physical health and sense of well being improved side by side, each bolstering the other and encouraging him to strive for even more.

As you move into a regular schedule of exercise, you will feel better about how you look and how you feel. While there is merit to the warning about being too prideful, an appropriate level of pride in your accomplishment will merely serve to inspire you to accomplish more. And if the goal of your efforts is physical, mental, and spiritual health, it would be difficult to determine a level where you have accomplished too much. After all, the closer you come to your old goals, the greater those goals become. The "best" you is probably beyond your imagining, but a better you is always within your grasp. You have only to make the decision to find it, and you will find it — every day!

The level of your interaction is equal to the level of your success.

— **Henry Ward Beecher**

THINKING THIN
Appendix 1
Your Body Mass Index

For those of you who are into math, here's a formula for figuring your Body Mass Index, courtesy of the National Institute of Health website.

$$BMI = \left(\frac{\text{Weight in pounds}}{\text{Height in inches}^2} \right) \text{ X } 703$$

For the rest of us, there's a table on the following page.

	Normal						Overweight					Obese					
BMI	19	20	21	22	23	24	25	26	27	28	29	30	31	32	33	34	35
Height (Inches)	Body Weight (pounds)																
58	91	96	100	105	110	115	119	124	129	134	138	143	148	153	158	162	167
59	94	99	104	109	114	119	124	128	133	138	143	148	153	158	163	168	173
60	97	102	107	112	118	123	128	133	138	143	148	153	158	163	168	174	179
61	100	106	111	116	122	127	132	137	143	148	153	158	164	169	174	180	185
62	104	109	115	120	126	131	136	142	147	153	158	164	169	175	180	186	191
63	107	113	118	124	130	135	141	146	152	158	163	169	175	180	186	191	197
64	110	116	122	128	134	140	145	151	157	163	169	174	180	186	192	197	204
65	114	120	126	132	138	144	150	156	162	168	174	180	186	192	198	204	210
66	118	124	130	136	142	148	155	161	167	173	179	186	192	198	204	210	216
67	121	127	134	140	146	153	159	166	172	178	185	191	198	204	211	217	223
68	125	131	138	144	151	158	164	171	177	184	190	197	203	210	216	223	230
69	128	135	142	149	155	162	169	176	182	189	196	203	209	216	223	230	236
70	132	139	146	153	160	167	174	181	188	195	202	209	216	222	229	236	243
71	136	143	150	157	165	172	179	186	193	200	208	215	222	229	236	243	250
72	140	147	154	162	169	177	184	191	199	206	213	221	228	235	242	250	258
73	144	151	159	166	174	182	189	197	204	212	219	227	235	242	250	257	265
74	148	155	163	171	179	186	194	202	210	218	225	233	241	249	256	264	272
75	152	160	168	176	184	192	200	208	216	224	232	240	248	256	264	272	279
76	156	164	172	180	189	197	205	213	221	230	238	246	254	263	271	279	287

THINKING THIN
Appendix 2
A Brief History of Hypnosis

The word "hypnosis" comes from the Greek word hypnos, meaning sleep. In Ancient Greece and Egypt, shrines and temples were built, where people were put in an induced sleep and given suggestions, which were thought to help healing.

It was not until the end of the 18th century, however, that the curative potential of these techniques was further explored and researched. In 1765, the Austrian physician Franz Mesmer put forward the theory that people could regulate the magnetism and fluids flowing through their bodies, and therefore play an active role in their own healing process.

In 1837, the English Professor of Medicine Dr. John Elliotson organized public demonstrations of mesmerism, shedding light on its effects on the muscular system. Ultimately, however, his work was discredited and Dr. Elliotson had to resign.

At the same time, the Scottish surgeon James Esdaile was using mesmerism as an anesthetic to perform operations on his patients in India, and reported a significantly lower rate of infection using this technique. However, his claims failed to convince the skeptical medical establishment.

The word hypnosis was used for the first time by British physician James Braid in the middle of the 19th century. Braid, rather than following Mesmer's magnetism theory, be-

101

lieved in stimulating the nervous system till exhaustion, in order to let his patients fall into a deep sleep, during which he would make some suggestions believed to cure them. After this, a number of doctors in Europe continued to move away from Mesmer's magnetism theory and use hypnotic suggestion to cure people. World War I served to spread hypnotism internationally, and a better understanding of the way the mind works facilitated this spread of knowledge.

Hypnotism reached the USA, where Milton Erickson brought it to another level when he found that hypnosis was a natural and spontaneous phenomenon, which we all experience frequently. By successfully demonstrating that hypnosis was not some unnatural phenomenon, Erickson helped to make it more mainstream and better accepted by the medical establishment. Around the same time, British physician Mason demonstrated to a group of fellow physicians the use of hypnosis in curing ichthyosis, a rare congenital skin disorder. Since that time, hypnosis has continued to spread and develop, and its uses and benefits have been demonstrated in a wider and wider range of fields.

In recent years, hypnotism, along with other alternative therapies, has become more mainstream every day. According to an article in the November 1997 issue of the Journal of the American Medical Association, there were more visits to alternative practitioners than to primary care physicians. The therapies which increased the most from 1990 to 1997 were herbal medicine, massage, vitamins, self-help groups, folk remedies, hypnotherapy, energy healing, and homeopathy.

Hypnosis is used medically as well as for behavior modification. The process assists to remove pre-operative anxiety and expedite post-operative healing, and is even used as natural anesthesia during operations. It has also been used to increase immune system efficiency, reduce nausea in chemotherapy patients, and much more.

Hypnotherapy has been mainly considered a behavior modification technique, rather than a natural extension of conventional medical treatment. However, if you realize that the subconscious mind literally runs the body, which as we know is the most complicated and efficient machine made, then it logically follows that we can direct the subconscious — through positive reinforced suggestions — to make the necessary changes the body needs to become healthy.

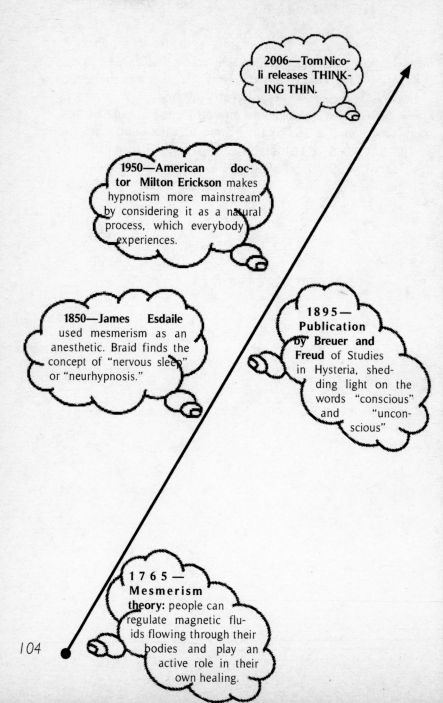

THINKING THIN
Appendix 3
Real People: Actual Results!

I am quite aware of the fact that there has been a flood of publicity about various weight loss programs these last few years, much of it riddled with claims of fantastic — and difficult to believe — results. While it's tempting to snicker and sneer at some of the come-ons, we need to keep in mind that they exist because of the genuine yearning so many people have to be thinner and more attractive.

Rather than quoting ad nauseam from studies written in such a way as to absolutely cure insomnia, I decided to share some actual, unedited feedback from just a few of my clients that reflect their feelings about the A Better You process. I will follow that with a couple of "composite case histories." To clarify this bit of doublespeak, a "composite case history" is a representative example of a typical individual's experience with my process, but is comprised of details gathered from several different individuals. This is done not to skew results in such a way as to make my process look more effective — which isn't necessary, anyway — but rather to more effectively ensure the privacy of individual clients. If you're working on losing weight, I'm sure you can understand how important that is.

It is my hope and intention that by showing you what people have written to me about their experience with hypnosis and weight loss that any fears and misgivings that you may have will be allayed so that you can procede with confidence to a new, better, and fitter you.

Dear Tom,

Three weeks ago, I met with you along with thirteen other women at an office in Melrose for a weight loss session. I have to say that, as a nurse, I was a little skeptical about how this would actually work. I thought that I would just let you know that so far, I'm very impressed. I have lost fourteen pounds in three weeks. It was always a struggle when I was doing Weight Watchers™. With hypnosis and listening to the CDs it has been much easier. Thank you so much.

Mark B.

Dear Tom,

I cannot tell you how many diets that I have been on and not many have worked. It's only been two weeks with your CDs and I have lost 12 pounds. That is great! I feel the best that I have felt in a long, long time, since about 10 years. Thanks again. Hope all is well with you and yours. Stay well and GOD bless you.

Di, Boston

Dear Tom,

Thank you so much for contacting me. Not only have I lost 35 pounds since the session, I lowered my blood pressure, which got me off my medication for a while now. I continue to listen to your CDs and am so grateful for the wonderful changes. Thank you so much!

Mary Ann, Malden, MA

Dear Tom,

I ordered the weight CDs from you a few weeks ago for myself, and it is working fantastically...I listen to it twice a day. First thing in the morning, and in the evenings before bed. I am eating much less, exercising much more, and I seem to have loads of energy...all that's thanks to you. Thank you again,

Suzanne S.

Hi Tom,

I recently purchased your weight loss CDs and love it. Not only is it relaxing me, but I think it's helping to calm my nerves too. I don't seem to have the problems with craving sugary items and junk food that had plagued me before. In addition to losing my ravenous desire for sweets and junk food, I've noticed that I am not as easily offended by others — things seem to roll off of me better. I'm waking up in a good mood and am feeling calmer and lighthearted throughout the day. This excites me because those are perks I hadn't even expected! I'm very much looking forward to buying more of your tapes. I'm so thankful to God for leading me to you!

Thanks for your help,

G. H., Sacramento, CA.

Hello Mr. Nicoli,

I purchased the weight loss CDs several weeks ago and have been using them daily for the last two weeks. Since then I have lost eight pounds with 15 to go. Of course I am thrilled!

Thank you,

Nel B.

Mr. Nicoli,

I received the CDs today and was very excited! I have listened to them several times already and am feeling great...I had a grilled Chicken Caesar salad for dinner (...one of my son had pancakes)... I am still awake, and have no desire for snacks, only water. YES!

Gettin' Slim in NY,

Leesa A.

Mr. Nicoli,

I ordered the C[...] and began on Saturday of this week. [...] impressed with CD 1 and started noticing changes in my eating behaviors immediately. Something must be getting through because I have lost seven lbs. in less than a week, and I feel wonderful.

Thank You,

Angie S.

These are but a few of the many letters I've received from people who have used my CD series or attended sessions I've conducted. Here are a couple of "composite case histories" I think you'll be able to relate to.

Brad's Story

"Brad" is a 31-year-old CPA from Milwaukee. He's not what you would call obese, but he has put on quite a few pounds since he finished grad school and got his accounting certification. He's a classic example of the guy who worked his way through an extended college education by working construction. He used to pride himself on his physique, which he kept up with long hours of manual labor. Once he entered the business world, however, his taste for physical exertion went away, but his taste for cheeseburgers remained intact. After only a few years of crunching numbers ten hours a day and crunching Quarter-Pounders™ the rest of his waking hours, his waist size was rapidly approaching symmetry with his age in dog years. The suits he had purchased at the beginning of his new career had all apparently shrunk dramatically (or at least, that's what he told himself). Ultimately, he had to admit that the clothes weren't shrinking...he was growing.

He made a real effort to replace his beloved hamburgers with salads, but always felt deprived by the substitution. And while he had good intentions when he signed the three-year contract with the gym, at the end of the day, the last thing he wanted to do was work up a sweat. To make matters worse, he felt embarrassed to present his growing paunch in the gym, which seemed to be populated with people more closely resembling Greek statues than everyday folks.

It seemed to Brad that he was doomed to his present state. He thought about using some of the diet drugs that were all the rage, until he started reading about people having heart attacks, strokes, and even "sexual side effects." He figured there was plenty of time for those, many years down the road. Then one day while surfing the Web, looking for an effective but safe way to lose a few pounds, he came across my website. He read every page — twice — before deciding to invest a few dollars in my Weight Loss CDs. He didn't really have much faith in my process, especially since it promised to make weight loss easy and painless. Brad had tried losing weight, and he knew better.

He listened to the tapes every day, and much to his surprise, after only a few weeks, he discovered that he had lost sixteen pounds. That was significant enough in and of itself. But what really shocked him was that when he took his girlfriend out to dinner one Friday night, he actually ordered grilled salmon and a vegetable medley rather than his usual steak and baked potato. It occurred to him that he had never ordered "girlie" food before, yet that night, it was what he craved. In addition to his mysteriously changing taste in food, he found himself actually looking forward to his thrice-weekly workouts, which had heretofore been a dreaded chore.

After just a few months, Brad had gotten his weight down to that of his college days. He also found that he felt more relaxed, got along better with co-workers and clients, and was generally more likeable. (Remember...he's a CPA. 'Nuff said.) While he started out with the clear, single goal of losing weight, he found that he was actually becoming a happier, healthier person, to boot. And he hasn't had a Quarter Pounder™ in months.

Footnote to Brad's story: I have absolutely nothing against any fast-food chain, and certainly have no intent to disparage McDonald's™ or their products. The simple truth is that, if you eat cheeseburgers — anybody's cheeseburgers — all the time, you're going to pack on the pounds, unless you have the metabolism of a hummingbird. Beef has fat in it. Period.

Ground beef has lots of fat. Eat enough of it, and you'll have fat in you, as well. It's simple physics. So send the lawyers back to doing whatever they do when they aren't suing people who talk about cheeseburgers, thank you.

Jennifer's Story

"Jennifer" is a forty-something mother of two, recently divorced and rediscovering the horrors of the singles scene. She has always been proud of her appearance, immaculate in her taste in clothes. She's one of those women who turn heads in a room when she enters. Since the divorce, however, she has come to the realization that she has put on a few pounds, and doesn't look as attractive as she would like in some of the new, more clingy fashions.

Having always been very health-conscious, Jennifer immediately ruled out diet pills as a means to lose weight, and simply wouldn't consider anything like liposuction. And what with the constant stress and demands of keeping up with two teenagers, a regular workout schedule just didn't seem feasible. Then, a friend of hers told Jennifer about my A Better You weight loss program and CDs.

Even though her friend spoke very highly of the process, Jennifer was quite naturally skeptical. To her, the whole hypnotism process just sounded too New Agey. But when her friend offered to reimburse Jennifer the cost of her consultation with me if it didn't work, she decided to give the process a try, figuring she had nothing to lose but the time spent listening to me.

Jennifer's initial reaction after our first session was that, while she did feel relaxed, there was nothing earth shaking about the experience. She decided to go ahead and come back a few more times, even though she doubted that the effort would have any real results. After a couple of sessions, however, she found that she was craving different foods than before. Where she had previously been addicted to anything that was smothered in Béarnaise sauce, she found that she now preferred a light vinaigrette. And while she had always indulged in the guilty pleasure of a second trip to the dessert cart after a sumptuous meal, she discovered that her once beloved French pastries no longer appealed to her.

She still didn't attribute her change in appetites to anything we did in our sessions, however. It wasn't until she found herself yearning for brisk rides on her bicycle, and found herself swimming vigorous laps in the health club pool, rather than languishing in the hot tub and sauna, that she realized that her preferences — indeed, her very lifestyle — were changing. She became aware of a newfound enjoyment of exercise, and although she certainly had not developed an aversion to the rich foods she had always craved, they simply bore little attraction to her any more.

Her new realizations inspired her to continue with the self-hypnosis exercises at home, and to begin monitoring her appearance more closely. After about a month, she began to notice that she was growing more fit. Her body seemed to have regained the tone it had in her youth, even to the point (it seemed to her) of defying what she had once thought to be the inevitable effects of gravity. When she finally weighed herself after six weeks, she found that she had only lost about five pounds. At first, she was disappointed, until she researched a bit. She learned that muscle is heavier than fat, and that it was not uncommon for people to actually look like they had lost weight when, in fact, they had remained the same or even gained a bit. The bottom line was that the mirror didn't lie; Jennifer looked and felt like she was ten years younger.

The only downside to her story (if you can call it a downside) is that Jennifer ended up spending considerably more than her regular clothing allowance, and she never asked her friend for the promised reimbursement. But, oh, what a difference! She honestly felt that she could give any of those young hotties a run for their money now. And she was right!

Though not everybody can expect to achieve the kind of results I have described in these examples, I feel certain that anyone who makes a conscious commitment to practice **THINKING** THIN will end up feeling better physically, and will discover that their general outlook on life will improve significantly. Those clients whose letters I've shared with you achieved noticeable results — and you can, too.

Furthermore, while this is what I do to earn my living, it is also a source of both great pride and humility that my efforts have been able to help so many people not only to overcome negative habits and behaviors, but to make dramatic improvements to their lives. And even though I certainly hope to sell a million or so copies of this book, my greatest hope is that even more people will find within the tools to make themselves happier and healthier.

I hope this book has given you a great start in reaching your goals. If, however, you think you would benefit from additional tools, don't miss the next section.

Appendix 4

Finding Additional Help

While a great many of you will find that the material presented in this book is sufficient to get you started on the path to losing weight and improving your health and general outlook, some of you will find that you respond more readily to being guided through the self-hypnosis process. It isn't that you lack the ability or intelligence to practice self-hypnosis; it's really more an issue of how you process information. Some people just respond better to guided imagery than to that which is created from their own experiences. Think of it as a matter of personality types and individual preferences.

Some people require, or simply prefer, one-on-one guidance to help them experience the benefits of hypnosis. I see thousands of these people each year in my private practice and seminar presentations. Although it is not particularly difficult to find a hypnotist, you will want to be sure that the practitioner you select is both qualified and proficient in addressing your specific requirements. Here are some guidelines you should follow in selecting the right person to work with.

Find the Right Person to Help You

- When seeking a hypnotist / hypnotherapist for personal change, it is important to ask questions. Never be shy

113

with any professional in any field. Asking questions is not only your right, it is your responsibility to yourself. So remember, when in doubt about anything, ask!

• Be sure the person is at least certified by a reputable organization. All organizations can be looked up on the Internet for validity. For example, I am certified with the National Guild of Hypnotists (NGH), the oldest and largest hypnosis organization in the world.

• What certifications do they hold, and how were the certifications obtained? CH or CHt designates a certified hypnotist/hypnotherapist. The National Guild of Hypnotists has higher levels of achievement, such as BCH (Board Certified Hypnotist).

• If working with a Ph.D., don't assume they must have extensive hypnosis training. I have found most do not, yet many will direct you away from any well-trained hypnotist/hypnotherapist.

• How long has the person worked in the field?

• More importantly, how many clients has this person worked with in that time? Some people work part time and have been in the field for 10 years, but have less actual experience with clients than someone who has been doing this for three to five years. For example, I did over 2,000 sessions in 2004 alone. Some people don't do that much work in five years.

• Has the practitioner worked with people in your specific situation? If the hypnotist or hypnotherapist you speak with works primarily with smokers and weight loss clients, and you are seeking relief from anxiety attacks or other physical disorders, you may want to find someone else.

• When working with any medical issue, always seek a physician's opinion first and ask for a referral for hypnosis work. Hypnosis sessions are not replacements for medical treatment, but are useful in conjunction with medical treatment.

- Does the individual you are considering have any testimonials available? People who succeed in any endeavor, especially one involving self-improvement, love to tell their stories. Any hypnotist worth his or her salt should have success stories available for your review.

- Finally — and just as important as any other qualification — you need to feel comfortable with the person you choose to work with. As with any type of partnership, the success of your efforts depends greatly upon how well you trust the other person. With hypnotism in particular, if you don't fully trust the hypnotist, you will never be able to relax your defenses enough to allow suggestions to take effect. A good rule of thumb is to ask yourself whether you would be comfortable sitting down to dinner with the person. If not, how could you expect to be comfortable allowing the person to enter your personal emotional space?

The National Guild of Hypnotists

The National Guild of Hypnotists, Inc. (www.ngh.net), with whom I hold my certification, is a not-for-profit, educational corporation in the State of New Hampshire. Founded in Boston, MA in 1951, the Guild is a professional organization committed to advancing the field of hypnotism. The Guild provides an open forum for the free exchange of ideas concerning hypnotism, highlighted during its annual conference. The Guild also provides resources for members, including certification programs, and the quarterly publication of the *Journal Of Hypnotism*™ and *Hypno-gram*™, and works as a vehicle for legal and legislative action.

Internet Resources

There are a number of entries on the subject of hypnotism in the online free encyclopedia Wikipedia. Here's a link to one of them you might find interesting: *http://en.wikipedia.org/wiki/Hypnosis*. At this website, you will find information on everything from the earliest history of hypnosis to modern applications.

If you type the word "hypnotism" into an Internet search engine, you will get listings for literally thousands of pages. Merely sorting the good sites from the bogus would be a daunting task, especially if you have a limited base of information upon which to make your determinations. The two sites noted above should provide you with answers to any questions you may have.

www.tomnicoli.com

THINKING THIN
Appendix 5
Hypnosis Audio Programs

Note: I am constantly adding to my product line, and prices are subject to change. For the most updated information please visit my website.

www.TomNicoli.com

Hypnosis Audio Programs — Complete Programs

The Ultimate Hypnosis Weight Loss System 6 CD Set
$87.77 (a $125 value)

> *The Original Weight Loss 2 CD set*
> *Carb Control Diet Plan 2 CD set*
> *Exercise Boost CD*
> *Subliminal Positive Reinforcement CD for Weight Loss*

Stop Smoking 5 CD Set
$72.77 (a $109 value)

> *Stop Smoking 2 CD set*
> *End Bad Habits CD*
> *Stress Releaser CD*
> *Subliminal Positive Reinforcement CD for Smoking Cessation*

The Emotional Freedom Series 6 CD Set
$95.77 (a $136 value)

Remove Emotional Clutter CD
Letting Go of the Past CD
Confidence Builder CD
Stress Releaser CD
Soothing Sounds CD for Meditation & Self Hypnosis
Subliminal Positive Reinforcement CD for Confidence & Self Esteem

The Executive Series 7 CD Set
$115.77 ($159 value)

Remove Emotional Clutter CD
End Procrastination & Self Limits CD
Increase Confidence & Self Esteem CD
Public Speaking Confidence CD
Stress Releaser CD
Goal Achiever CD
Subliminal Positive Reinforcement CD for Increased Confidence

Stress Management 4 CD Set
$59.77 ($91 value)

Stress Releaser CD
Goal Achiever CD
Confidence Builder CD
Subliminal Positive Reinforcement CD for Confidence & Self Esteem

Academic Peak 5 CD Set
$72.77 ($109 value)

Academic Peak 2 CD set - Remove test anxiety while building better study habits, faster reading ability, improved memory and retention, and more...
Confidence Builder CD
Goal Achiever CD
Subliminal Positive Reinforcement CD for Goal Achieving

Athletic Improvement Series 6 CD set
$89.77 ($130 value)

> *Athletic Performance Improvement I - Overall Athletic Improvement*
> *Athletic Performance Improvement II - Mind Practice Guided Imagery & Visualization*
> *Confidence Builder CD*
> *Goal Achiever CD*
> *Exercise Boost CD*
> *Subliminal Positive Reinforcement CD for Increased Confidence*

Golf Confidence 5 CD Set
$76.77 (a $114 value)

> *Golf Confidence CD*
> *Athletic Performance Improvement II- Mind Practice Guided Imagery & Visualization*
> *Confidence Builder CD*
> *Goal Achiever CD*
> *Subliminal Positive Reinforcement CD for Goal Achieving*

TOM **NICOLI**

Hypnosis Audio Programs — 2 CD Sets
Each 2 CD Set is $39.77 (a $45.54 value)...

Weight Loss
Carb Control
Stop Smoking
Athletic Improvement
Academic Peak

Single CD Hypnosis Helpers
Each CD in this list is $22.77...

Exercise Boost
Goal Achiever
Confidence Builder
Stop Self Sabotage
End Bad Habits
Letting Go of the Past
Remove Emotional Clutter
Stress Releaser
End Procrastination & Self Limits
Golf Confidence
Public Speaking Confidence
Soothing Sounds for Meditation & Self Hypnosis

To purchase online, please visit *www.TomNicoli.com*.

Name: _____

Mailing Address: _____

City: _____

State: _____ Zip: _____

Payment: (circle one)   Check   Credit Card   **Only Visa and MC, please!**

Credit Card #: _____

Exp.: _____ 3-digit Code: _____

Signature: _____

Item Name	Quantity	Price	Total

Total amount of order	$
Shipping	$5.00
Total	$

Mail this order form and payment to:
A Better You Hypnosis, Inc.
400 West Cummings Park
Suite 1350
Woburn, MA 01801

All hypnosis audio CDs have a 30-day, no questions asked personal satisfaction guarantee. If they aren't exactly as I've described them or you aren't satisfied with the results you achieve after following the exercises, I'll buy the CDs back from you!

About the Author

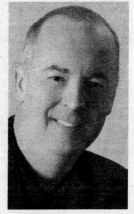

Award-winning, Board Certified Hypnotist Tom Nicoli is a published author, public speaker, expert witness, trainer and innovator in the industry of hypnotism.

Nearing his 20th anniversary as an internationally trained Hypnotist, Tom's practice has helped clients from every walk of life tackle some of life's most complex behavioral and physical challenges with profound results.

Nicoli has successfully treated more 10,000 people with a 98% success rate throughout his nearly 20 years' experience. His clients typically seek relief from a personal issues including but not limited to simple behavioral challenges, addictions, weight loss, motivation, and chronic emotional and physical disorders.

A contributing author to a variety of publications and adjunct faculty member of the National Guild of Hypnotists (NGH), Nicoli is a dynamic seminar leader and lecturer, with frequent expert guest appearances on television and radio programs worldwide including *NBC News*, *Dateline NBC*, *Talk of the Town*, *The Jordan Rich Show*, and the popular Massachusetts cable television show *Healthy Hypnosis*. Tom Nicoli owns and operates **A Better You Hypnosis, Inc.** in Woburn, MA, where he conducts private sessions. His vast clientele includes professional athletes, celebrities, and international royalty, from locations spanning the globe throughout the US, Switzerland, Dubai, Europe, and Canada.

KALLISTI

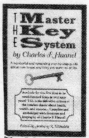

The Master Key System
Charles F. Haanel

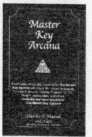

Master Key Arcana
Charles F. Haanel
& others

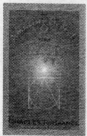

**The Amazing Se-
crets of the Yogi**
Charles F. Haanel

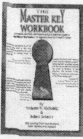

**The Master Key
Workbook**
Tony Michalski
& Robert Schmitz

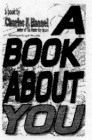

A Book About You
Charles F. Haanel

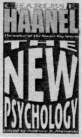

The New Psychology
Charles F. Haanel

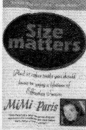

Size Matters!
MiMi Paris

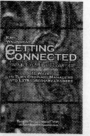

**Getting Connected
Through Exceptional
Leadership**

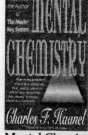

Mental Chemistry
Charles F. Haanel